The Lidcombe Program of Early Stuttering Intervention

The Lidcombe Program of Early Stuttering Intervention

A Clinician's Guide

Mark Onslow

Ann Packman

Elisabeth Harrison

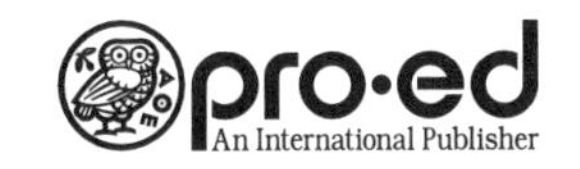

8700 Shoal Creek Boulevard
Austin, Texas 78757-6897
800/897-3202 Fax 800/397-7633
www.proedinc.com

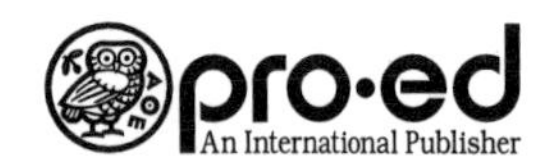

© 2003 by PRO-ED, Inc.
8700 Shoal Creek Boulevard
Austin, Texas 78757-6897
800/897-3202 Fax 800/397-7633
www.proedinc.com

Library of Congress Cataloging-in-Publication Data

The Lidcombe program of early stuttering intervention : a clinician's guide / Mark Onslow, Ann Packman, Elisabeth Harrison.
p. cm.
Includes bibliographical references and index.
ISBN-13: 978-089079904-8
ISBN-10: 0-89709-904-0
1. Stuttering in children. 2. Stuttering in children—Treatment. I. Onslow, Mark. II. Packman, Ann. III. Harrison, Elisabeth.

RJ496.S8 L53 2002
618.92'855406—dc21 2002068051

This book is designed in Goudy and Frutiger.

Printed in the United States of America

4 5 6 7 8 11 10 09 08 07

Contents

Preface

The prime motivation for the preparation of this text was to relieve us of the repetitive task of providing basic information about the Lidcombe Program during clinical training. The Lidcombe Program of early stuttering intervention is a parent-conducted, behavioral treatment for stuttering, designed for children younger than 6 years of age. Not only does this book provide basic information about the program but it contains nearly all the detailed information about it that we can think of at present. As such, it is adequate to serve as a reference manual for clinicians who use the treatment.

We use the term *clinicians* throughout the book to refer to those qualified professionals whose job titles are speech pathologists, speech–language pathologists, speech–language therapists, and so on. It is for them, and students of this profession who are destined to join them, that we prepared this book. Nevertheless, this text is in no way intended to constitute a thorough clinical training. In our view, nothing can replace mentorship in the development of clinical competence with this treatment.

The compilation of this text is not meant to imply any finality in the development of the Lidcombe Program. However, at this time we believe that published outcome data are sufficiently compelling to justify some confidence in the procedure. We do not know who will complete the job of assembling an adequate evidence base for the Lidcombe Program, or when it will be completed. We certainly intend to participate in that endeavor, but we know that it will probably take more time than we have.

The writing of this book occurred shortly after the 10th anniversary of the first report of the treatment that was later to be called the Lidcombe Program. During the celebrations of that anniversary in 2000, in communicating with those who had been associated with the project, it became apparent to us how popular the treatment had become around the world. We are not sure why that is so. Perhaps the Lidcombe Program has tapped a vein of clinical common sense. We would like to think that its popularity also has something to do with its links to scientific principles, in both its origins and its continued development.

Some thanks are due. First, thank you to our chapter authors for their nearly always cheerful tolerance of our demands. If we have achieved nothing else, perhaps it is an entire work in the English language that does not have a single incorrect use of the apostrophe. Thanks also to Martin Wilson and Peggy Kipping at PRO-ED, who have been nothing but helpful and supportive throughout, and to Giri Hegde for his gentle corrections to our potential damage to the English language.

Final thanks go to Roger Ingham, whose influence in the development of the Lidcombe Program has been acknowledged in these pages. It was he who led us to take for granted the importance of scientific principles in any satisfactory treatment for stuttering and showed us how that could be achieved. Without that, we do not think the Lidcombe Program would have been possible. So, our final keystrokes dedicate this book to Roger John Ingham.

Mark Onslow
Ann Packman
Elisabeth Harrison
Sydney, Australia
November 2001

Contributors

Cheryl Andrews, MSc
Children's Hospital Medical Centre
Sydney, Australia

Joseph Attanasio, PhD
Montclair State University
Upper Montclair, New Jersey
United States

Marjorie Blakeley, DipTchg
Stuttering Treatment and Research Trust
Auckland, New Zealand

Rebekah Dredge, BAppSc
Children's Services, The Spastic Centre
Metropolitan South and West Region
Sydney, Australia

Joan Girson, BA
Department of Speech Pathology and Audiology
University of the Witwatersrand,
Johannesburg, South Africa

Barry Guitar, PhD
University of Vermont
Burlington, Vermont
United States

Vanessa Harris, MAppSc
Stuttering Unit, Bankstown Health Service
Sydney, Australia

Elisabeth Harrison, BAppSc
Stuttering Unit, Bankstown Health Service
Sydney, Australia

Rosemarie Hayhow, MSc
United Bristol Healthcare Trust and Speech & Language Therapy Research Unit, Frenchay Hospital
Bristol, United Kingdom

Sally Hewat, BAppSc
Australian Stuttering Research Centre
The University of Sydney
Sydney, Australia

Mark Jones, BSc
Clinical Trials Research Unit
The University of Auckland
Auckland, New Zealand

Mary Kingston, BA
Norwich NHS Primary Care Trust
Norwich, United Kingdom

Rebeccah Ledzion, BSpPath
Smooth Talk Ltd.
Cambridge, United Kingdom

Caron Levy, BA
Department of Speech Pathology and Audiology
University of the Witwatersrand
Johannesburg, South Africa

Michelle Lincoln, PhD
School of Communication Sciences and Disorders
The University of Sydney
Sydney, Australia

Margaret Marks Wahlhaus, PhD
Australian Stuttering Research Centre
The University of Sydney
Sydney, Australia

Sue O'Brian, BAppSc
Australian Stuttering Research Centre
The University of Sydney
Sydney, Australia

Mark Onslow, PhD
Australian Stuttering Research Centre
The University of Sydney
Sydney, Australia

Tika Ormond, BSc
Department of Speech and Language Therapy
University of Canterbury
Christchurch, New Zealand

Ann Packman, PhD
Australian Stuttering Research Centre
The University of Sydney
Sydney, Australia

Isabelle Rousseau, MHSc
Australian Stuttering Research Centre
The University of Sydney
Sydney, Australia

Rosalee Shenker, PhD
The Montreal Fluency Centre
Montreal, Quebec
Canada

Kerry Ttofari, BSpPath
Department of Education and Training
Melbourne, Australia

Margaret Webber, MSc
Stuttering Unit, Bankstown Health Service
Sydney, Australia

JoAnne Wilding, MSc
The Montreal Fluency Centre
Montreal, Quebec
Canada

Linda Wilson, BAppSc
School of Community Health
Charles Sturt University
Albury, Australia

Part I

Background

Chapter 1

Overview of the Lidcombe Program

Mark Onslow

This text is designed to be a comprehensive clinical primer for the Lidcombe Program of early stuttering intervention, as well as a source of information about its background and its use at various locations around the world. The purpose of this chapter is to provide the reader with a fundamental reference point for using the text. Here, the nature of the treatment and its fundamental concepts and procedures are overviewed, along with the body of empirical literature that supports it.

Before proceeding, however, it is worthwhile to expand on one component of the previous paragraph: the concepts and procedures of the Lidcombe Program. This treatment is not a set of programmed, predetermined procedures. To those who have written this book, it is axiomatic that there are as many different ways of doing the Lidcombe Program as there are children who stutter and their families that receive the treatment. In other words, *the Lidcombe Program is individualized for every child and family.* Understanding of this notion is the entry-level understanding for using the treatment.

What Kind of Treatment Is the Lidcombe Program?

A Treatment Developed by Clinicians and Researchers

The Lidcombe Program was developed in the Sydney suburb of Lidcombe, in a collaboration between researchers at The University of Sydney and professional clinicians at the Stuttering Unit, Bankstown Health Service, Sydney. It was not developed solely within a university. We believe this is one of the reasons that clinicians have accepted the program in Australia and are doing so increasingly around the world (see Part IV). The procedures described in this text have their current form after years of trial and fine-tuning by clinicians who specialize in stuttering. This fine-tuning process began in Lidcombe Hospital and was continued at the Stuttering Unit. What is written about in this book is what clinicians can do as a part of their everyday caseloads, and what they enjoy doing every day. All of the clinical outcome data about the Lidcombe Program that we consider at the end of this chapter were collected during the course of the daily practices of clinicians in public clinics in Australia.

It also bears stating that the Lidcombe clinics in which this treatment developed are not elite in any sense of the word. To the contrary, Lidcombe is a middle to low socioeconomic suburb, as is Bankstown, where the Stuttering Unit it currently located. The clinics are public, not private, being funded by the taxpayer, so clients do not pay a fee for service. Lidcombe and Bankstown are multicultural suburbs, with many residents who do not speak any English, and consequently many of the treatment sessions are conducted with the aid of an interpreter. Also, the Stuttering Unit attracts many difficult-to-treat stuttering preschool children (see Chapter 10) because it has gained a reputation as a specialist clinic. As such, many problematic cases are referred there for management from the Sydney metropolitan areas, when clinicians have not successfully brought stuttering under control.

A Behavioral Treatment

The Lidcombe Program is a behavioral treatment in that its focus is on the problem behaviors of stuttering. My colleagues and I (Harrison, Onslow, Andrews, Packman, & Webber, 1998) have pointed out that, in the case of adults who stutter, in only some cases is it viable for a treatment to be focused exclusively on the *problem behaviors* of the condition; much more is at stake in the management of chronic stuttering in adults than the control of stuttered speech. However, we know of no reason at present to believe that, when presented with a preschool child who has begun to stutter, a clinician needs to do anything more than eliminate stuttered speech—in other words, to restore the perception to all that the child has normally developing speech, as was the case before the onset of the disorder. Everything that occurs in the Lidcombe Program is focused on getting rid of the incipient problem behaviors of stuttering in preschool children. *The goal of the Lidcombe Program is, simply, no stuttering.* The research overviewed later in this chapter suggests that this goal is realistic and attainable.

It is worth clarifying the terminology we use for stuttering at this point. The Lidcombe Program incorporates the concept of a "moment of stuttering." Although there are many issues surrounding this notion (for a review, see Onslow, 1996), we have found it suitable for clinical practice and outcome research. During the Lidcombe Program, and throughout this text, moments of stuttering are referred to using the terms *stutter, stuttering,* or *stuttered.* As described in Chapter 6, when we talk about stuttering to children, we use various terms (e.g., *bumpy*). We prefer not to use *dysfluency, nonfluency,* and their variants such as *dysfluent* and *nonfluent,* because they are indirect. The Lidcombe Program is about behavioral control of stuttering, so we refer to stuttering with terms that relate directly to the problem behaviors of concern. In referring to speech that does not contain stuttering, we use the term *stutter-free* rather than *fluent,* again because it is direct and relates to the problem behaviors that are the focus of treatment. With children, we use terms such as *smooth* to describe stutter-free speech (see Chapter 6).

A Treatment Developed for Children Younger Than 6 Years

The Lidcombe Program was developed for children younger than 6 years, and this text deals with its application to that age group. This does not mean that it cannot be applied to older children. In fact, it has been shown to be effective for children from 7 to 12 years of age (Lincoln, Onslow, Lewis, & Wilson, 1996). It is clear from that research, however, that overall the treatment is not quite as effective with children in that age range as with children younger than 6 years. It would seem that, with increasing age, this style of treatment becomes less effective. File audits of the Lidcombe clinics in Sydney show many instances when 7- and 8-year-old children respond to the treatment in the same way as younger children, but the Lidcombe Program alone appears to be insufficient to eliminate stuttering in some children in the 7- to 12-year age range. In essence, we know little about this issue at present, and consequently treatment of children older than 6 years is beyond the scope of this text.

A Treatment Implemented by Parents

The Lidcombe Program is not conducted by the clinician; it is conducted by parents. The role of the parent is to do the treatment in the child's everyday environment, and the role of the clinician is to teach the parent to do the treatment. The only time the clinician does the treatment is to demonstrate it for the purposes of teaching parents.

Most likely, this is one of the reasons why outcome data for the Lidcombe Program have been so favorable (as discussed later in this chapter): The treatment happens where the problem happens. Children stutter during everyday speaking situations, and the treatment happens in those situations. As such, generalization of treatment effects with the Lidcombe Program is not an issue, because there is nothing to generalize! This is one of the reasons why it is critical that the clinician does not do the treatment; doing so, in effect, introduces the issue of generalization. In other words, when treatment effects occur in the clinic, they must generalize beyond the clinic for the treatment to be effective. Apart from the risk of complicating the treatment by introducing generalization, the notorious risk of discriminated learning with this disorder (Ingham, 1984; Onslow, 1996) makes it potentially detrimental for the clinician to do any of the treatment. One of the worst things for a clinician to hear when treating stuttering children—heard all too often with clinic-based treatments for older children—is a parent report that the child does not stutter in the clinic but does so beyond the clinic.

In conducting workshops around the world, the Lidcombe clinicians often state that clinicians are experts in how to treat early stuttering, but parents are the experts with their children. The Lidcombe Program draws on that expertise that parents have about their own children; they know what they like, they know what they do not like, they know what motivates them best, and so on. Most important, they have special relationships with their children. Treatment differs from family to family, but, for the most part, the parent–child relationship is always there and it is the task of the clinician to incorporate that relationship into the Lidcombe Program. This is why the Lidcombe Program is done differently with every family: because every parent–child relationship is different.

The incorporation of the parent–child relationship into treatment is one of the reasons why the Lidcombe Program is enjoyable for parents and children. The parent and child do it together, and together they control the stuttering. Interviews with parents who have treated their children show this (see Chapter 16). Although parents can initially be apprehensive using the procedures, eventually the treatment is associated with a sense of accomplishment, and they feel empowered having done it. It is much the same for the children. Parents tell us that children welcome the treatment, and even prompt their parents to do it on occasions when parents forget. In general, the Lidcombe Program is a treatment that children and parents enjoy. If this enjoyment does not occur, then, simply, it does not work. These points are well illustrated in the parents' comments about the treatment in Chapter 16.

What Is the Treatment Agent in the Lidcombe Program?

In short, the treatment agent is parental verbal contingencies for stutter-free speech and stuttered speech, during everyday life. Stutter-free speech and stuttered speech are the two so-called responses of the Lidcombe Program. To say that parental verbal contingencies occur for a child's responses means that, after stutter-free speech or stuttered speech occurs, parents may say certain things. Those certain things—the parental contingencies—are acknowledging the response, praising the response, and asking the child to self-correct the response.

A full discussion is in Chapter 6, but in summary, the procedure works as follows: On some occasions during everyday life together, parents acknowledge when their children have stutter-free speech, and at other times, praise them for stutter-free speech. On still other occasions, parents acknowledge a moment of stuttering. On some of the latter occasions, a parent may choose to ask the child to repeat the utterance without the stuttering. In other words, the parent asks the child to self-correct stuttered speech. To guarantee that the treatment is a positive experience for the child, a rule of thumb in the Lidcombe Program is that there should be at least five times the amount of acknowledgment and praise for stutter-free speech as there is the acknowledgment and asking for self-correction of stuttering. In short, the fundamental treatment procedure of the Lidcombe Program is parental verbal contingencies for responses during everyday conversations. From that concept its procedures emerge, (and again we stress) the implementation of which always differs from family to family.

When the Lidcombe Program was first publicized beyond Australia in the mid-1990s, we encountered recurring expressions of concerns that parents were "correcting" their child's stuttering (e.g., Onslow, O'Brian, & Harrison, 1997). Obviously, this concern was associated with a lasting influence of the diagnosogenic theory of stuttering onset[1] (for overviews, see Chapter 3; Onslow, 1996). We always found this concern bemusing because, in reality, a parent correcting a child's speech makes no clinical sense at all. It is not the parent who corrects the child's stuttering in the Lidcombe Program, but the child. What the parent does is to ask the child to correct a stuttered utterance. The parent only asks the child to do that in an appropriate and supportive manner, and at an appropriate and well-chosen time and place.

The Lidcombe Program has no other treatment agent apart from parental verbal contingencies. This is what controls the stuttering. Another way of saying this is that stuttering in small children is an operant. The Lidcombe Program does not involve rate control or any adjustment to the child's customary way of speaking. Furthermore, the Lidcombe Program does not demand any adjustments to the child's living environment in the belief that features of the environment are the cause of stuttering, of its perpetuation, or both. Such notions are at the heart of multifactorial treatment models for early stuttering, such as the demands and capacities model (for an overview, see Chapter 3). Certainly, the Lidcombe Program involves minor changes in children's daily living environments. But those changes are simply that parents present contingent verbal stimulation to control stuttering. Unlike treatment prompted by the Demands and Capacities model, the Lidcombe Program is atheoretical, to the extent that it does not derive its procedures from a theory of the nature or cause of stuttering in children.

[1] Obviously attributable to the same source is another recurring concern about discussing early childhood stuttering in a clinic with the child present. We still find that many clinicians, particularly in the United States, find this to be something that they do not routinely do in a speech clinic.

At this stage in the overview of the Lidcombe Program, two points warrant highlighting. The first is that, although it can be a clinical challenge, what the clinician is trying to achieve is fundamentally simple. Parents essentially praise children and draw attention to stuttering and sometimes ask for self-correction. The essentials of the treatment are not complicated. The second point is that the parental verbal contingencies must not be constant, intensive, or invasive. If they are, the results will be disastrous. It is not difficult to imagine a child's response if parents commence unremitting negative input contingent on every moment of stuttering. The Lidcombe Program requires parents to be extremely selective about when they provide verbal response–contingent stimulation to their children. In particular, it is clinical disaster if those contingencies impair the child's everyday communication with parents. As stated, the Lidcombe Program draws on the special relationship between parents and children, and it is critical that its procedures do not cause any kind of deterioration in that relationship. These and other topics relating to common problems with the Lidcombe Program are addressed in Chapter 8.

How Is the Lidcombe Program Implemented?

The basic method of service delivery with the Lidcombe Program is that the child and parent(s) visit the clinic each week as the clinician trains the parent(s) to implement the procedures. In practice, we find that morning or early afternoon is the best time to schedule appointments for preschool children. In the experience of the Lidcombe clinicians, more often than not one parent attends the clinic each week with the child, although both parents participate. On some occasions, significant other people in the child's life also participate. As the treatment progresses, the clinician teaches different things to the parent. This is fundamental to the treatment; as the child improves, the parents have to learn new skills. *Doing the same thing each week when the parent and child visit the clinic is a sign that things are not going well.*

As mentioned and reiterated already, the treatment is individualized for each child, and there are as many individual presentations of the Lidcombe Program as there are families with a stuttering preschooler who come to a clinic for help. This is so important: The treatment relies absolutely on the relation between parents and child, and every such relationship is different, as is every child and every parent. Consequently, every presentation of the Lidcombe Program is different. However, as noted previously, in each case the clinician is attempting to achieve the same thing: parental verbal-contingent stimulation of various responses during everyday conversations.

A treatment that includes verbal contingencies for stuttered speech invokes a duty of care for the clinician. Because, as noted, it is potentially problematic if this procedure is done incorrectly, the clinician needs to ensure that parents are presenting verbal contingencies safely and correctly. Therefore, at the start of the Lidcombe Program, when the parent is first learning to give various verbal contingencies, the parent does so in carefully structured conversations only. This initial structured application of verbal contingencies facilitates the initial teaching of the parent by the clinician of the basic procedures of the treatment. Furthermore, consistent with standard clinical practices, it enables the parent to ensure that the task is organized flexibly so that the child's responses are mostly correct. Finally, structured parental verbal contingencies at the start enable the child to get used to the treatment, and enable the parent to convey positive and helpful messages to the child about what is occurring. When the parent has mastered the requisite skills, and the child is happy with the procedure, parental verbal contingencies in everyday, unstructured situations are introduced.

Measurement of stuttering is part of the Lidcombe Program, and is considered in detail in Chapter 5. At the start of each clinic visit, the clinician makes an objective measure of the child's stuttering severity that is based on a count of the number of stutters that occur during conversation. But more important, each day the parent uses a simple and convenient 10-point severity rating scale to record the child's stuttering severity. These measures enable the clinician and parent to communicate effectively about the child's stuttering, so that they both know how severe it is, and when and where it is most and least severe. Furthermore, within- and beyond-clinic measures provide the critical information for the Lidcombe Program: Is the treatment working? The only way to really know this is with comprehensive beyond- and within-clinic speech measures (see Chapter 5). It is so important to know whether the treatment is working, because, if it is not, the reason needs to be established and rectified. This is particularly important during the first weeks of treatment. Speech measures during the Lidcombe Program guide management decisions, and without them it is simply not possible to do the treatment correctly. Failure to collect and correctly interpret and clinically respond to speech measures is a source of one of the major problems in implementing the Lidcombe Program, and this topic is covered in detail in Chapter 8.

The Two Stages of the Lidcombe Program

The Lidcombe Program is implemented in two stages. In Stage 1, the goal is for the child to have no stuttering in everyday speaking situations, and Stage 1 concludes when stuttering reaches predetermined low criteria. At this point, speech measures assume another integral part in the treatment: They are used to specify exactly what the child's speech must be like for Stage 1 to have been considered a success. There is nothing vague about this. It is a precise process, and the benefits of that precision are realized during Stage 2 of the treatment. Speech measures continue during Stage 2, and are used to determine whether the child is continuing to maintain treatment benefits. During Stage 2, the family visits the clinic less frequently if the child maintains treatment benefits, and eventually they stop visiting altogether.

Historically, stuttering has been thought to be a relapse-prone disorder. Stage 2 of the Lidcombe Program corresponds to what might be termed "maintenance" in other treatments. We prefer not to use that term, because it implies that the treatment is finished, whereas this is far from the case with the Lidcombe Program. Stage 2 is an inherent part of the program; it is not something that is added to the conclusion of treatment, as occurs in some other stuttering treatments. During Stage 2, the parent gradually withdraws the verbal contingencies, and gradually assumes complete responsibility for the treatment as visits to the clinic decrease in frequency. Any departure from the criterion speech performance, as specified with the clinical measures at the end of Stage 1, is actioned immediately. This important phase of the treatment is considered in detail in Chapter 7.

Figure 1.1 overviews the implementation of the Lidcombe Program. Box 1.1 overviews the key concepts and procedures of the Lidcombe Program presented so far.

A Typical Clinic Visit with the Lidcombe Program

To give the reader a feel for what the Lidcombe Program is like, the following is a description of the usual way clinic sessions are conducted when the parent and child attend each week. Although this sequence is varied by the Lidcombe clinicians according to need, on most occasions the following sequence happens.

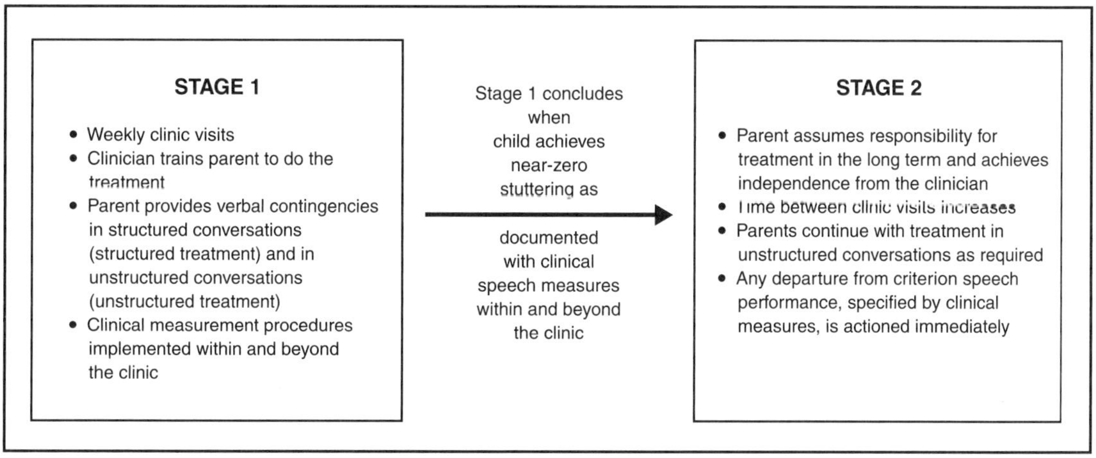

STAGE 1

- Weekly clinic visits
- Clinician trains parent to do the treatment
- Parent provides verbal contingencies in structured conversations (structured treatment) and in unstructured conversations (unstructured treatment)
- Clinical measurement procedures implemented within and beyond the clinic

Stage 1 concludes when child achieves near-zero stuttering as documented with clinical speech measures within and beyond the clinic →

STAGE 2

- Parent assumes responsibility for treatment in the long term and achieves independence from the clinician
- Time between clinic visits increases
- Parents continue with treatment in unstructured conversations as required
- Any departure from criterion speech performance, specified by clinical measures, is actioned immediately

Figure 1.1. Overview of the Lidcombe Program of early stuttering intervention.

Box 1.1

Key Concepts and Procedures of the Lidcombe Program Presented So Far

- The Lidcombe Program is a behavioral treatment with a goal of no stuttering.
- It is not a programmed set of procedures.
- The Lidcombe Program is driven by concepts.
- The treatment happens where the problem happens.
- The treatment agents include praise for stutter-free speech and acknowledging and asking for self-correction of stuttered speech.
- Parental verbal contingencies are not constant, intensive, or invasive.
- Parents and children enjoy the treatment and find a sense of accomplishment in it.
- The treatment is done by the parents in everyday life situations.
- The clinician does not do any treatment but, in the clinic each week, trains the parent to do the treatment.
- The parent is taught new procedures each week as the treatment progresses.
- The treatment draws on parents' expertise with their own children.
- There are as many different ways of doing the treatment as there are families with a stuttering child.
- The treatment happens in structured conversations before occurring in everyday, unstructured conversations.
- Clinical measurement is inherent and essential in the Lidcombe Program, being the basis for its operation.
- The goal of Stage 1 is no stuttering, and the goal of Stage 2 is for parents to maintain treatment effects in the long term, with increasing independence from the clinician.

The first procedure on arrival is for the clinician to make an objective measure of stuttering severity while talking to the child, while watching the parent talk to the child, or a combination of both. Then, the parent presents severity ratings for the child's stuttering on each day during the previous week, and the parent and clinician compare the clinician's measure in the clinic and the parent's measures outside the clinic. Inherent in this discussion is the consideration of progress during the previous week: whether the child's stuttering is decreasing and how the parent has managed with the treatment. The latter topic is discussed in-depth, so that any problems with implementing the treatment can be uncovered. Progress is impeded if there are any problems that the clinician fails to identify. Then, the parent demonstrates the treatment procedures that were used at home during the previous week, and the clinician gives the parent feedback. Then, the clinician explains to the parent what changes will be implemented during the coming week, and demonstrates those changes to the parent. Subsequently, the clinician trains the parent to do the changed procedures, giving feedback and demonstrating as needed. In concluding the session, the clinician summarizes what the parent is to do when conducting the treatment during the coming week, and encourages the parent to ask questions to clarify any matters.

The Evidence Base for the Lidcombe Program

Inherent in a behavioral treatment is the reliance on scientific clinical research for treatment procedures. Therefore, being a behavioral treatment, the Lidcombe Program depends on scientific evidence for its credibility and for its development. There are a number of sources of such evidence. Fundamentally, for its procedures, it draws on laboratory evidence of the ameliorative effects of contingent stimulation on stuttering, which is overviewed in Chapter 3. For more direct evidence of its effectiveness, it draws on a number of outcome studies that have been published to date. These studies all carry the methodological and accepted credentials of being based on reliable, objective measures of speech, during everyday childhood situations, for a clinically meaningful period post-treatment. These studies are summarized in Box 1.2 and Figure 1.2. At the time of writing, a randomized controlled trial is in progress (Jones, Gebski, Onslow, & Packman, 2001). This is the "gold standard" of clinical trials, and permits conclusions about the efficacy of the treatment. At present, our outcome data allow only a confident statement that children are not stuttering when assessed after the treatment. Those data do not permit conclusions about whether the treatment provides effects beyond those of natural recovery.

Nonetheless, while we wait for completion of the current randomized controlled trial, we feel that confidence in the treatment is justified, for three reasons (Onslow & Packman, 2001). First, there are outcome data to show that stuttering is at near-zero levels in school-age children after the treatment (Lincoln et al., 1996). This age group has little chance of natural recovery, which suggests that it is the treatment that is responsible for this effect. Second, the known predictors of the rate of recovery with the Lidcombe Program are different from those known to be indicative of whether or not natural recovery will occur (see Onslow & Packman, 2001). Third, a recent experiment by Harris, Onslow, Packman, Harrison, and Menzies (in press) showed that over a 12-week period, stuttering children who received the Lidcombe Program improved more than stuttering children who did not.

The other type of research that supports the Lidcombe Program deals with the process of the treatment rather than the outcome of the treatment: Treatment process research. This line of inquiry focuses not on measures

Box 1.2

The following outcome studies all incorporated reliable, objective speech measures of stuttering rate beyond the clinic in everyday childhood speaking situations, and were conducted over a clinically meaningful period. A detailed overview of the methods in these studies can be found in Onslow, Menzies, and Packman (2001).

- *Onslow, Costa, and Rue (1990)*: A preliminary report of the procedure with four children. Data appeared to show a promising trend of recovery after the treatment, which lasted for 9 months.
- *Onslow, Andrews, and Lincoln (1994)*: A first attempt at having a control group in order to study the effects of the treatment against the effects of natural recovery. The control group could not be maintained, with the parents opting to "drop in" to the treatment group rather than having treatment withheld. In effect then, this study was an outcome study of 12 children who received the Lidcombe Program. The results showed that this group was virtually not stuttering 12 months after the treatment, in a variety of everyday childhood speaking situations.
- *Lincoln and Onslow (1997)*: A long-term follow-up study of 42 children who received the Lidcombe Program. Results showed that, at 4 to 7 years posttreatment, stuttering remained at near-zero levels in everyday speaking situations.

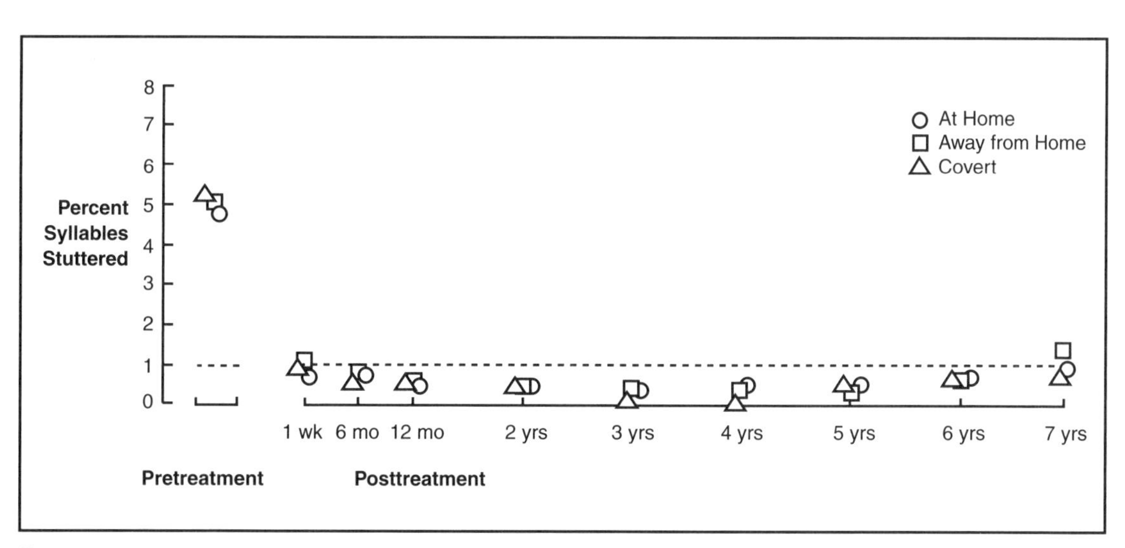

Figure 1.2. Summary of available outcome data for the Lidcombe Program at the time of writing. These data points summarize the data described in Box 1.2. Data are presented for the percentage of syllables stuttered by the children while talking at home and outside their homes, and also for covert assessments when the children were not aware that their speech was being recorded. *Note.* Adapted from "Long-Term Outcome of an Early Intervention for Stuttering," by M. Lincoln and M. Onslow, 1997, *American Journal of Speech–Language Pathology*, 6, p. 56. Adapted by permission of the American Speech-Language-Hearing Association.

designed to capture what is thought to be a desirable treatment outcome, but on measures that are designed to convey information about how the treatment works. The earliest treatment process study, by Lincoln, Onslow, and Reed (1997), was essentially a social validity study, which showed that children's speech posttreatment was perceptually indistinguishable from that of control children. This study provided the fundamental information that the Lidcombe Program treatment process is different from adult treatments that produce their effects by inducing a novel and unusual sounding speech pattern. Exactly how the Lidcombe Program works is not known at present. However, some preliminary studies have provided no reason to believe that the treatment induces extensive change in language function of the children or of their parents (Bonelli, Dixon, Bernstein Ratner, & Onslow, 2000) or that the treatment induces extensive changes in speech acoustics (Onslow, Stocker, Packman, & McLeod, 2002). The Lidcombe Program introduced a novel procedure to speech–language pathology practices with small children; hence, it was important to demonstrate that there is no reason to believe that it causes anxiety or a problem with the parent–child attachment (Woods, Shearsby, Onslow, & Burnham, 2002).

Probably the most important treatment process research with the Lidcombe Program to date was that of Jones, Onslow, Harrison, and Packman (2000). They demonstrated with 250 children that the median time required to meet the program criterion of near-zero stuttering was 11 visits by the parent(s) and child to the clinician. This figure of 11 clinic sessions seems robust, because it replicated what was found by the Lidcombe research teams in Australia (Onslow et al., 1994) and the United Kingdom (Hayhow, Kingston, & Ledzion, 1998). Jones et al. also reported the shape of the recovery plot for the Lidcombe Program and an analysis of the capacity of case history variables to predict treatment time. This study, and other treatment process studies, are summarized in Boxes 1.3 through 1.7.

In summary, treatment outcome and process research has provided sufficient evidence to warrant confidence in the outcome of the Lidcombe Program. Treatment process research has provided data to suggest that the treatment is safe, and has provided benchmark data that can be used by clinicians who use this treatment. The remainder of this text is a detailed exposition of the methods of the Lidcombe Program, with case studies, a consideration of its inherent issues, and the experiences of clinicians who have used it in various countries. Appendix 1.A supplements treatment overview by providing information that was assembled from

Box 1.3

Lincoln, Onslow, and Reed (1997) conducted a study of the social validity of the Lidcombe Program outcome data. The first part of the study compared posttreatment stuttering measures of a group of children who had been treated with the Lidcombe Program and a group of control children. No differences were found between the groups. The second part of the study compared the number of "stuttering" versus "not stuttering" judgments made by experienced clinicians and unsophisticated listeners for the two groups. Findings showed that unsophisticated listeners could not distinguish between the treated and the control group with these perceptual methods.

Box 1.4

Multifactorial models such as the Demands and Capacities model (see Chapter 3) suggest that one explanation for the favorable outcome data with the Lidcombe Program might be that there is comprehensive shutdown or simplification of nontargeted language function in children and their families. Bonelli, Dixon, Bernstein Ratner, and Onslow (2000) studied the language of 8 children and their mothers before and after the Lidcombe Program. Pretreatment and posttreatment measures of child and parent speech rate, interspeaker turn latencies, and pragmatic functioning revealed no patterns that might account for treatment effects. In fact, results showed that maternal speech rate increased in posttreatment speech samples and the mothers reduced the proportion of their utterances in which they requested information from their children. Another important finding in the data was that all the children's language measures were within or above appropriate developmental levels. These results ruled out the possibility, as suggested by the Demands and Capacities model, that the Lidcombe Program curtails language functioning in families.

Box 1.5

Several theoretical perspectives on early stuttering suggest that the direct methods of intervention in the Lidcombe Program may be associated with negative psychological effects on children and on the relationships between children and their parents. The most notable of these is the now discredited diagnosogenic theory. In response to a variety of published concerns about possible harm to children arising from the Lidcombe Program, Woods, Shearsby, Onslow, and Burnham (2002) sought evidence of systematic and pernicious effects on a group of children over the pretreatment to posttreatment period. The *Child Behavior Checklist* (CBCL; Achenbach, 1988, 1991) is a tool designed to detect in children behavioral signs of anxiety, aggression, withdrawal, or depression. "Attachment" is a construct relating to the bond between parent and child, and is thought to be developmentally important in early childhood. The *Attachment Q-Set* (AQS; Waters, 1995) is a tool for measuring the quality of the attachment relationship between child and mother. Over the pretreatment to posttreatment period, neither of these measures provided any evidence of a systematic deterioration of any psychological construct. If anything, the results for the CBCL were consistent with posttreatment improvements. These results are consistent with a view that the Lidcombe Program is a safe treatment for children and their families.

detailed observations of Lidcombe Program clinic visits. These are records of only a few visits, so they describe only a few of the events that might occur during a visit. In other words, the appendix is not a complete record of everything that might occur during clinic visits, but a sample of what might occur.

Box 1.6

A common treatment approach to the control of stuttered speech in adults is the use of a novel and frequently unusual sounding speech pattern. Research has shown that these changes in speech motor functioning during treatment are associated with measurable changes in the timing of acoustic segments. Most commonly, reports show that measures such as vowel duration, voice onset time, and intervocalic interval increase after treatment when stuttering is controlled. This information raises the possibility that the Lidcombe Program prompts children to make changes to their habitual speech motor functioning, perhaps subtle changes that have not been obvious to their clinicians. To investigate this possibility, Onslow, Stocker, Packman, and McLeod (2002) made various measures of acoustic segment timing over the pretreatment to posttreatment period in a group of children being treated with the Lidcombe Program. No evidence was found for any consistent and systematic effects that might provide an explanation for the effects of the treatment in terms of changes to speech motor functioning.

Box 1.7

There is a chance that any child who comes for treatment shortly after stuttering onset will recover naturally. Therefore, the timing of early intervention is an important consideration for clinicians. They must decide between waiting to see if natural recovery might occur, and controlling stuttering immediately by intervening with the Lidcombe Program. Jones, Onslow, Harrison, and Packman (2000) sought to establish information that might be relevant to clinicians about this issue, by seeking case history predictors of requisite treatment time for 250 children who were successfully treated with the Lidcombe Program. Logistical regression methods were used to explore whether treatment time could be predicted by gender, age, onset-to-treatment period, and stuttering severity. Results showed no relation between age or onset-to-treatment intervals and treatment times. In other words, in children younger than 6 years, a short delay before beginning treatment with the Lidcombe Program appears not to make the condition less tractable. If anything, the data suggested that very young stuttering preschool children might not respond as quickly to the treatment as older preschool children. It is critical to note that these results pertain only to children younger than 6 years, and the results cannot be extrapolated to older children. In fact, outcome data for older children (Lincoln, Onslow, Wilson, & Lewis, 1996) suggest that the outcomes for older children with the Lidcombe Program are considerably less favorable than for children younger than age 6. An additional aspect to the Jones et al. article was that it established some important benchmarks. The median treatment time for the 250 children to complete Stage 1 was 11 clinic visits, and the shape of the recovery plot for the Lidcombe Program was presented. This recovery plot is reproduced in Figure 1.3. At present, the shape of the recovery plot for natural recovery is unknown, but this will be important information to be established in the future, to assist clinicians in the timing of early intervention.

(*continues*)

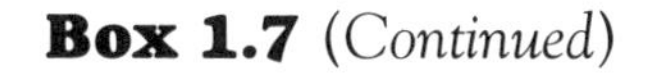

Box 1.7 *(Continued)*

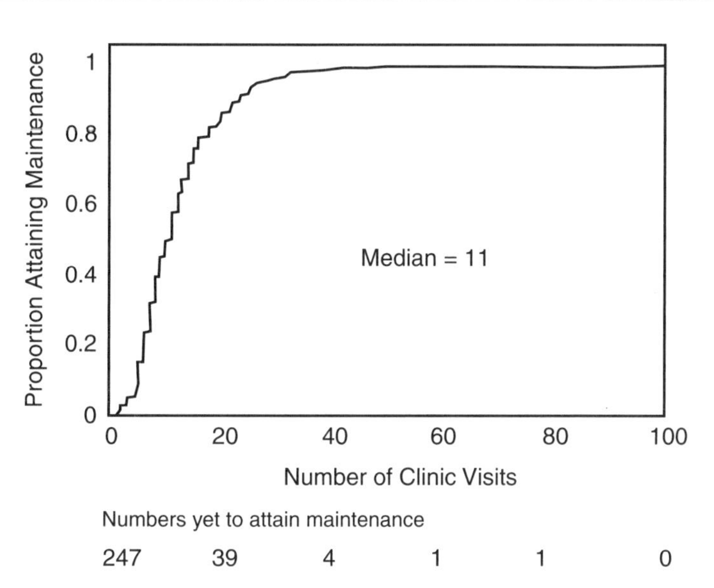

Figure 1.3. Recovery plot showing number of clinic visits required to complete Stage 1 by 250 children treated with the Lidcombe Program. *Note*. From "Treating Stuttering in Children: Predicting Outcome in the Lidcombe Program," by M. Jones, M. Onslow, E. Harrison, and A. Packman, 2000, *Journal of Speech, Language, and Hearing Research, 43*, p. 1446. Copyright 2000 by the American Speech-Language-Hearing Association. Reprinted with permission.

Appendix 1.A

Sampling of Events from Lidcombe Program Clinic Visits

The following list outlines what the clinician might do during a typical Lidcombe Program clinic visit.

Introduction

Greets child and parent

Supplies child with activity or toy
- tells child how to use activity or toy
- talks about activity or toy with child
- joins in play or activity

Tells child what will happen next during the clinic visit

Tells parent what will happen next during the clinic visit

Within-Clinic Speech Sampling

With parent, engages child in conversation
- asks child to select activity, toy, or book from a closed set
- provides child with toy, activity, or book
- converses with child
- repeats child's utterances
- expands on utterances

Informs parent
- about expectations of within-clinic speech sample
- that within-clinic speech measures may not be representative of the child's usual speech
- about requirements of the speech sample
  - required length
  - spontaneous conversation

Provides parent with observations about the speech sample
- child is talking a lot
- compares amount of talking to previous week
- describes types of stuttering
- compares types of stuttering with previous visit
- describes general severity of stuttering
- compares severity of stuttering to previous visit

Collecting Background Information

Asks parent about treatment conducted during previous week
- type of treatment (e.g., in structured or unstructured conversation)
- how often (e.g., twice daily)
- for how long

Asks parent about aspects of child's stuttering
- compares within- and beyond-clinic severity ratings (SRs)
- compares current and past SRs
- considers whether there is any pattern to fluctuations in stuttering
- considers whether there are certain circumstances under which child stutters severely
- gives examples of such situations

Beyond-Clinic Tape Recording

Provides parent with
- information about
  - beyond-clinic requirements
    - —why a tape-recorded sample is required
    - —duration of tape recording
    - —number of tape recordings to be done in the following week
  - observations from a beyond-clinic tape recording of child since previous visit (i.e., general severity)
- praise and encouragement for making beyond-clinic tape
- written instructions of what is required from beyond-clinic tape recording

Ensures parent has tape recorder available

Responds to parent's queries or concerns about difficulties with tape recording and provides suggestions
- on contexts in which to take tape recordings

- to overcome difficulties (e.g., leave tape recorder visible all the time to desensitize the child to it, allow child to play with tape recorder)

Within-Clinic Speech Sample

Introduces button-press event counter
- tells child that event counter will be used
- allows child to push buttons on event counter
- tells child that event counter will be used to count child's words

Measures percentage of syllables stuttered (%SS) on-line with event counter with child in clinic

Provides parent with
- information about
  - number of stutters in within-clinic sample
  - observations from within-clinic measures (e.g., compares %SS to previous visit)
  - the need for parent participation in counting stutters from beyond-clinic sample
- speech measures
  - results of within-clinic sample
  - results of beyond-clinic sample

Requests that parent count the number of stutters on the beyond-clinic recording

Severity Ratings (SRs)

Provides parent with information about
- rationale for comparing clinician's and parent's SRs (i.e., to ensure reliability)
- how to assign a severity rating
  - record maximum SR for the day
  - make several ratings in various contexts
  - assess for a specific period per day
- fluctuations in SRs
  - they are common
  - they can be sign of progress
- measures
  - clinician's SR for within-clinic sample
  - comparison between clinician's and parent's SRs

Provides praise and encouragement to parent
- for collecting SRs
- for SR given to within-clinic sample

Gathers information
- asks parent for SR for within-clinic speech sample
- asks parent for SRs collected since last clinic visit
- asks parent if SRs reflect child's overall speech throughout the week
- writes parent's SRs into clinic file notes
- requests daily SRs for beyond-clinic situations until next clinic visit

Responds to parent's request for clarification about how to assign SRs

Giving Parents Information About Stuttering

Provides parent with information about
- what is stuttered speech by illustrating difference between stuttered speech and normal disfluency in a tape-recorded sample
- fluctuations in stuttering (i.e., stuttering may increase under some circumstances)
  - when child is tired
  - when child is excited
  - during spontaneous speech

Responds to parent's enquiry about
- the nature of stuttering
- whether there is a relationship between stuttering and talking fast

Encouraging Parent–Client Cooperation

Asks parent
- generally
  - if there are any questions
- specifically
  - if there are any concerns about
    —doing treatment
    —collecting speech measures

Provides parent with
- information about clinic visit proceedings (i.e., what will happen next during the clinic visit)
- information about concentration span (i.e., appropriate expectations for the age of the child)
- praise and encouragement
  - for information supplied
  - for asking questions and making comments by saying that concerns and questions are normal

Gives child
- praise about proceedings
  - what will happen next during the clinic visit
  - that the event counter will be used
  - that child can play with activity or toy
- praise and encouragement for activities or play
  - verbally
    - —by giving suggestions for activity or play
    - —by acknowledging child's talking during play
  - tangibly

Requests acknowledgment and approval from child
- to talk to parent
- about what will happen next during the clinic visit

Treatment

Gives parent information about
- general topics
  - importance of keeping treatment positive
  - the way to administer treatment to the child
    - —structured or unstructured conversations
    - —when
    - —how often
    - —where
  - rationale for the way treatment will be administered to the child
  - techniques for eliciting the desired type of speech
- treatment in unstructured conversations
- rationale
  - that verbal contingencies should only relate to stutter-free speech and stuttering
  - that most of the time no verbal contingencies are given
- treatment in structured conversations
  - what treatment will involve
    - —low-key verbal contingencies
    - —positive verbal contingencies
  - duration
  - flexible treatment practices
    - —to increase amount of stutter-free speech when SR is high
    - —to stop when child shows signs of losing interest
- what is required of child
  - to talk with SR of 1 to 2
  - to self-correct stuttered words
- praise
  - supplementing praise with activities during structured conversations
  - when to give the praise
    - —when child talks smoothly
    - —intermittently
- beyond-clinic requirements
- treatment outcome
  - illustrates probable outcome using other clients' SR charts (i.e., patterns that tend to occur during treatment)
  - explains that unusual behaviors used to control stuttering are not part of the treatment
- criteria to enter Stage 2
  - estimation of when this will occur
  - variable as each child is different

Provides parent with praise and encouragement
- for doing treatment at home
- for the way the parent has conducted treatment

- for suggesting rewards to use during treatment
- by giving specific feedback about parent's treatment

Collects information about
- whether treatment was done during previous week
- outcome of treatment as agreed during previous clinic visit
- frequency of verbal contingencies used per day or hour
- child's response to treatment

Responds to parent's concerns or queries about
- treatment in unstructured conversations
- what treatment to do in the week ahead
- variable severity of child's stutter

Demonstrates treatment in structured conversations by engaging child in conversation
- asks child to select activity or toy from a closed set
- withholds parts of toy or activity
- provides child with toy or activity
- asks child question about toy or activity
- makes comments about toy or activity
- converses with child
- asks parent to encourage child to talk

Provides child with information about
- requirements of treatment
  - stutter-free speech
  - self-correction of stuttered speech
- activities and toys (i.e., child will receive a piece of the toy or activity when speech is stutter-free)

Provides child with verbal contingencies during demonstration of treatment in structured conversation
- tells child he or she said a smooth sentence or word
- tells child that he or she is talking smoothly
- tells child that he or she is saying stuttered words smoothly when asked to repeat them
- requests child to self-correct stuttered word
  - with model
  - without model

Asks parent to demonstrate treatment in the clinic

Praises parent
- for giving effective verbal contingencies
- for giving specific feedback

Summing Up

Provides parent with date and time for next clinic visit

Informs child that it is time to finish clinic visit

Plans for next clinic visit
- asks child and parent to bring in toy or activity for next clinic visit
- asks child what toy or activity clinician should bring to next clinic visit

Requests child's approval to pack away toys and activities

Thanks child for coming

References

Achenbach, T. M. (1988). *Child behavior checklist for ages 2–3*. Burlington: University of Vermont.

Achenbach, T. M. (1991). *Manual for the child behavior checklist/4–18 and 1991 profile*. Burlington: Department of Psychiatry, University of Vermont.

Bonelli, P., Dixon, M., Bernstein Ratner, N., & Onslow, M. (2000). Child and parent speech and language and the Lidcombe Program of Early Stuttering Intervention. *Clinical Linguistics and Phonetics, 14,* 427–446.

Harris, V., Onslow, M., Packman, A., Harrison, E., & Menzies, R. (in press). An experimental investigation of the impact of the Lidcombe Program on early stuttering. *Journal of Fluency Disorders*.

Harrison, E., Onslow, M., Andrews, C., Packman, A., & Webber, M. (1998). Control of stuttering with prolonged speech: Preliminary outcome of a one-day instatement program. In A. K. Cordes & R. J. Ingham (Eds.), *Treatment efficacy for stuttering: A search for empirical bases* (pp. 191–212). San Diego: Singular Publishing Group.

Hayhow, R., Kingston, M., & Ledzion, R. (1998). The use of clinical measures in the Lidcombe Programme for children who stutter. *International Journal of Language & Communication Disorders, 33,* 364–369.

Ingham, R. J. (1984). *Stuttering and behavior therapy: Current status and experimental foundations*. San Diego: College-Hill Press.

Jones, M., Gebski, V., Onslow, M., & Packman, A. (2001). Design of randomized controlled trials: Principles and methods applied to a treatment for early stuttering. *Journal of Fluency Disorders, 26,* 247–267.

Jones, M., Onslow, M., Harrison, E., & Packman, A. (2000). Treating stuttering in young children: Predicting treatment time in the Lidcombe Program. *Journal of Speech, Language, and Hearing Research, 43,* 1440–1450.

Lincoln, M., & Onslow, M. (1997). Long-term outcome of an early intervention for stuttering. *American Journal of Speech–Language Pathology, 6,* 51–58.

Lincoln, M., Onslow, M., & Reed, V. (1997). Social validity of an early intervention for stuttering: The Lidcombe Program. *American Journal of Speech–Language Pathology, 6,* 77–84.

Lincoln, M., Onslow, M., Lewis, C., & Wilson, L. (1996). A clinical trial of an operant treatment for school-age children who stutter. *American Journal of Speech–Language Pathology, 5,* 73–85.

Onslow, M. (1996). *Behavioral management of stuttering*. San Diego: Singular Publishing Group.

Onslow, M., Andrews, C., & Lincoln, M. (1994). A control/experimental trial of an operant treatment for early stuttering. *Journal of Speech and Hearing Research, 37,* 1244–1259.

Onslow, M., Costa, L., & Rue, S. (1990). Direct early intervention with stuttering: Some preliminary data. *Journal of Speech and Hearing Disorders, 55,* 405–416.

Onslow, M., Stocker, S., Packman, A., & McLeod, S. (2002). Speech segment timing in children after the Lidcombe Program of early stuttering intervention. *Clinical Linguistics and Phonetics, 16,* 21–33.

Onslow, M., Menzies, R., & Packman, A. (2001). The Lidcombe Program: Development of a parent-conducted operant early intervention for stuttering. *Behavior Modification, 25,* 116–139.

Onslow, M., O'Brian, S., & Harrison, E. (1997). The Lidcombe Programme: Maverick or not? *European Journal of Disorders of Communication, 32,* 261–266.

Onslow, M., & Packman, A. (2001). The Lidcombe Program of early stuttering intervention: Awaiting the results of a randomised controlled trial. *Asia-Pacific Journal of Speech, Language, and Hearing, 6,* 85–89.

Waters, E. (1995). Appendix A: The Attachment Q-Set (version 3.0). In E. Waters, B. E. Vaugh, G. Porsada, & K. Komdo-Ikemura (Eds.), Caregiving, cultural, and cognitive perspectives on secure-base behavior and working models: New growing points of attachment theory and research. *Monographs of the Society for Research in Child Development,* 60(Serial No. 244), pp. 234–246.

Woods, S., Shearsby, J., Onslow, M., & Burnham, D. (2002). The psychological impact of the Lidcombe Program of early stuttering intervention: Eight case studies. *International Journal of Language & Communication Disorders, 37,* 31–40.

Chapter 2

From Laboratory to Living Room: The Origins and Development of the Lidcombe Program

Mark Onslow

My co-contributors to this text wished for a short record of the history of the Lidcombe Program to be among its opening chapters. Being the only member of the original Lidcombe Program team who remains at Lidcombe, the Sydney suburb where this treatment has developed over the years, I was nominated for the task. Now that this treatment is becoming popular around the world (see Part IV), it might be an appropriate time to briefly record some history. In short, academicians at a campus of what was to become The University of Sydney, in the Sydney suburb of Lidcombe, worked closely with clinicians at the Stuttering Unit at Lidcombe Hospital, in the development of the Lidcombe Program. Many things have changed, but we are still teaching about the treatment and working on it, and publishing papers. But how and why did we all get here? The story begins in the early 1970s, and I want to tell aspects of it that cannot be found in any of our publications to date. More important, I want to acknowledge the contribution of some people in the development of the treatment who have not figured in our publications. My history ends in 1990, the date of the first publication dealing with the procedure.

The Lidcombe Program is a product of places, people, and times that crossed paths on two continents over three decades. In this short history, I trace those times, people, and places that constitute the history and background of this treatment. In effect, verbal response-contingent stimulation as a means to control the stuttering in preschool children found its way from the experimental laboratory of the University of Minnesota into the living rooms of parents of stuttering children who use the Lidcombe Program today. That development constitutes the finding of a clinical model for the application of verbal response-contingent stimulation to the problem of early stuttering. In essence, that is what the Lidcombe Program is: a clinical model adapted from a scientific laboratory model. The start of the development of this model was in Minnesota.

Minnesota, United States

It was the early 1970s. During the previous two decades, researchers had established that stuttering could be brought under laboratory control with operant methods. Those methods included activities that were not clinically usable, such as shock and loud noise, so I suppose that is why it was some time before anyone took it many steps further and tried to make these operant methods work for children.

Not that anyone would have wanted to, because Wendell Johnson's (Johnson et al., 1942) diagnosogenic theory was accepted at the time and everyone thought that to do anything operant with preschool children would be a clinical error that would worsen the problem. It would be 11 years before Prins and Ingham (1983) published their seminal text, in which the authorities of the day publicly renounced Johnson's theory and advocated direct treatment of early stuttering. And it would be 14 years before Oliver Bloodstein—Johnson's disciple—published his statement that it was clinically impossible to convince parents of stuttering children that the only problem was their own behavior (Bloodstein, 1986). It was a time when the idea of directly controlling a child's stuttering was light years away. But the method to do so was there in the results from an American research laboratory. The place was the University of Minnesota, which housed the world's finest operant research lab for stuttering. The people were Richard Martin,[1] Gerald Siegel, and Samuel Haroldson. Also there was a relatively unknown Australian psychologist, from Sydney, by the name of Roger Ingham, who was visiting the University of Minnesota as a postdoctoral student. He rejoins the story a few years later.

The merits of great ideas cannot be judged in isolation as the achievements of those who had them. They need to be judged also in the context of the time and place in which they occur. In that context, one would be hard pressed to find a better example of a research idea in our field than the one behind the so-called puppet study (Martin, Kuhl, & Haroldson, 1972). Martin et al. devised an ingenious method to apply operant laboratory findings on stuttering to preschool children. A talking puppet was mounted and illuminated in a box, and the experimental children sat in a room and conversed with the puppet (a.k.a. Patricia Kuhl). The puppet was operated from outside the room by the experimenters. A baseline period involved a number of 20-minute conversations with the puppet, which the child enjoyed. Then, each time the child stuttered, the experimenters turned out the light for a few seconds, effectively making the puppet "disappear." After a short time, the light came back on and the child and puppet continued their conversation.

And there you have it—a key factor in the origins of the Lidcombe Program. Not far from the cradle of the diagnosogenic theory in Iowa, at a time when nobody could bear to think about operant methods with preschoolers, these researchers, who had given shock and loud noise to stuttering adults, devised a gentle and creative way to present experimental operant methods to young stuttering children. Most significantly, their results were spectacularly successful. The two experimental children stopped stuttering in the Minnesota lab while talking to Suzybelle, the puppet, and generalized those gains to outside the clinic, and still showed those gains a year later. Tragically, one of the children was killed in a car accident 12 months after the experiment finished. The other is now an adult living somewhere in the United States. For ethical reasons, his identity and location are unavailable. But I would not be surprised if he is not stuttering and, as appears to be the case with children who have a successful treatment for stuttering in early childhood (see Chapter 16), has forgotten all about the stuttering in his past.

Considering the context in which it was conducted, the puppet study was quite challenging to prevailing beliefs, to say the least. Many years later in Sydney, some indication of that challenge found its way to me during a conversation with Jerry Siegel. Jerry had been a part of the Minnesota research team, though not directly involved in the puppet study. As it happened, he also had been a doctoral student at the University of Iowa, and had been profoundly influenced by Wendell Johnson (who,

[1] Shortly after the preparation of this text, we were saddened to hear news of the death of Richard Martin on October 26, 2001.

from all accounts, was a charismatic man). One day in Lidcombe we were watching a video of myself demonstrating some of the techniques in the Lidcombe Program with a 3-year-old child, and he said that he winced every time I drew attention to stutteing. It just went completely against every clinical instinct he had with preschool stuttering children, even though he had been in the research setting where the puppet study had generated such convincing evidence of the therapeutic properties of the procedure. I found this to be revealing about the depth of influence of the diagnosogenic theory, and how challenging the puppet study was to it.

Sydney, Australia

So, how does the development of the Lidcombe Program switch from Minnesota to Sydney, Australia? Remember that quite unknown psychologist, Roger Ingham, who was at Minnesota when the puppet study was conducted? Well, he did not remain unknown for long. On route to that prominence, and many other distinctions, Roger found his way to Lidcombe. In 1972 he was appointed head of the School of Communication Disorders in what was eventually to become part of The University of Sydney. His interest in stuttering sustained not only his own career, but those of many who came in contact with him. Some of those were the original developers of the Lidcombe Program, which included myself.

Roger Ingham's influence on the Lidcombe Program is extensive. When using the treatment around the world today, clinicians do things that derive directly from his influence. For example, they measure stuttering severity within and beyond the clinic, and they incorporate those measurements into management. Also, the procedures for maintenance of treatment effects in the Lidcombe Program (see Chapter 7) are based directly on his experimental work. But for the way things happened to work out during his first days in Sydney, Roger's influence in treatment of early stuttering may have been not only extensive, but also direct. Indeed, it might have been he who developed the Lidcombe Program, or something like it.

In 1972, Roger Ingham's thoughts turned to a replication of the puppet study. This occurred in a speech clinic in a Sydney hospital. He had a puppet system installed and began to run one subject, with one of the staff providing the puppet's voice. The experiment failed because, according to Ingham, the child's "stuttering simply diminished to zero during base rate. But I then got hung up with other projects and never returned to children" (personal communication, November 4, 1999). Included among those other projects was his research program into prolonged-speech treatment for adults. As the topic of his doctoral thesis, prolonged speech was Ingham's major career interest at that time. The rest of that is in the history of the development of treatments for adults, but Ingham never returned to treatment research with children.

For the rest of the 1970s, clinical interest in the puppet technique languished, even though its results were replicated to some extent with other reports (e.g., Reed & Godden, 1977). During the 1980s I heard one report of a clinician in Sydney attempting the procedure. Also, during the 1980s I saw a video of a university clinician working with a puppet apparatus. For my part, in 1976 I crossed paths with Roger Ingham professionally when he was my academic teacher in stuttering at what was called at the time Cumberland College of Health Sciences.

When I received my first job as a clinician in a Sydney hospital, one of the first things I did was to ask my department head, Robyn Murrell, if I could try the puppet technique. She did not think that a puppet was the answer to stuttering in children but gave me her support, even though her specialist clinician in stuttering at the time was philosophically horrified by the idea of using operant methods with stuttering preschoolers, and even though a department of child and family psychiatry, located down the hall, supervised our department's treatment of stuttering and found the whole thing abhorrent. The intellectual freedom Robyn Murrell gave me in 1980 contributed to the development of the Lidcombe Program.

I had the hospital carpenters build a puppet theater with an open front that was pressed against the outside of a one-way window into my clinic room. The theater had a light that illuminated the puppet, which I could operate with a foot switch. A microphone sent my assortment of puppet voices (my favorite was Woofa the dog) into the room where the child sat and, along with me, had a terrific time. When the child stuttered, out went my foot, out went the light, and the puppet disappeared. So there I was for many hours in the darkened corridor outside my room talking to children with funny puppet voices. Robyn Murrell was right. A puppet is not the clinical solution to stuttering in preschoolers. Close, but not quite right. What the puppet study really says did not occur to us until many years later.

My days as a clinician came to an end when I was offered a job at the School of Communication Disorders at Cumberland College of Health Sciences, in Lidcombe, where Roger Ingham was located. I accepted the job, and Roger Ingham's influence on me there resulted in a lifelong enthusiasm for working with stuttering. In 1985 Roger Ingham left Lidcombe to take up a post at the University of California, Santa Barbara. That left me as the academician in the department responsible for the area of stuttering. Ingham had done so much with adults, so I decided that I would work with children. I returned to the task of finding out how the puppet study could be used as the basis of a treatment of early stuttering.

Finding out how to do that turned out to be quite a long project. First came the idea that the parents could be Suzybelle, and they could be Suzybelle during everyday life instead of in a laboratory or a clinic, and that would do away with problems with generalization, because the treatment could happen where the problem of early stuttering happens. Much to my regret, the first two Australians to use the Lidcombe Program to my knowledge—or at least a primitive version of it—never made it into any publication on the topic. They were Miriam Potter and Deborah Morris, two of my clinical students who attempted to have parents do a "Suzybelle." I acknowledged their input into our work in a forgotten publication from that time, which I consider to be the first published documentation that foreshadows the Lidcombe Program.

Once we stumbled onto the idea of having parents do a variant on what Suzybelle did, we were on the right track. The treatment is verbal response-contingent stimulation, and the treatment model is to have the parents do it. That model evolved over several years with clinical trial and error, evaluated with clinical outcome measures. Initially, there was excitement when it seemed to work for a few children, and then puzzlement when it did not work for many others. During 1984, Leanne Costa, Cheryl Andrews, and I founded the Stuttering Unit, which was staffed jointly by Lidcombe Hospital and the School of Communication Disorders.[2] The Stuttering Unit was the place where the Lidcombe Program continued its original development. We all worked for a few years figuring out why our techniques did not work for some kids. In those years we stumbled across things that we now take for granted about the Lidcombe Pro-

[2] The foundation of the Stuttering Unit was possible because of the cooperation and goodwill from Anne Deane, who was head of the Lidcombe Hospital Speech Pathology Department at the time, and Joan Rosenthal, who was acting head of the School of Communication Disorders at the time. Also, the Stuttering Unit could not have existed without the support of Drs. Carter and Miller, superintendent of Lidcombe Hospital and principal of Cumberland College, respectively. The Stuttering Unit is now located near Lidcombe in the Sydney suburb of Bankstown.

gram, such as—parents do not need to make a fuss, that treatment has to be supportive, that parents need to use praise more often than they request self-correction, that parents need to measure the child's speech, and so on—all the features of the treatment we describe in this book. The effective elements started to become apparent in the period from 1984 to 1988, as we experimented clinically at the Stuttering Unit. Eventually, the clinical data that we used to evaluate our attempts at refining the treatment began to show consistent results. Gradually, parents began to tell us consistently the positive stories that we report in Chapter 16, and gradually we began to settle into the clinician behaviors of the Lidcombe Program that we record in Chapter 1.

In 1988 we were sufficiently confident in the treatment to begin work on our first data-based outcome study, which was published some time later (Onslow, Costa, & Rue, 1990). That publication began the phase of the procedural development that is on record in the literature, and that is where this background ends.

References

Bloodstein, O. (1986). Semantics and beliefs. In G. H. Shames & H. Rubin (Eds.), *Stuttering then and now* (pp. 130–139). Columbus, OH: Merrill.

Johnson, W., et al. (1942). A study of the onset and development of stuttering. *Journal of Speech Disorders, 7*, 251–257.

Martin, R. R., Kuhl, P., & Haroldson, S. (1972). An experimental treatment with two preschool stuttering children. *Journal of Speech and Hearing Research, 15*, 743–752.

Onslow, M., Costa, L., & Rue, S. (1990). Direct early intervention with stuttering: Some preliminary data. *Journal of Speech and Hearing Disorders, 55*, 405–416.

Prins, D., & Ingham, R. J. (Eds.). (1983). *Treatment of stuttering in early childhood: Methods and issues*. San Diego: College-Hill Press.

Reed, C. G., & Godden, A. L. (1977). An experimental treatment using verbal punishment with two preschool stutterers. *Journal of Fluency Disorders, 2*, 225–233.

Chapter 3

The Lidcombe Program in Historical Context

Barry Guitar

The Lidcombe Program is, in many ways, a radical departure from previous approaches to stuttering in preschool children. It can also be seen, however, as descending from an old tradition of direct treatment of early childhood stuttering. This chapter supports and expands both of these perspectives, giving some historical background for the Lidcombe Program and illuminating its differences and similarities with other approaches.

One of my motivations for writing this chapter is that I have seen many children benefit from the Lidcombe Program. A number of clinicians in the United States, however, have been opposed to it, some even calling it the devil's work. I hope to reduce a little of the resistance to the Lidcombe Program by reminding readers that many of the procedures have been used successfully by parents and clinicians for decades. Even the most controversial elements of the program, such as having parents correct moments of stuttering, have been used—albeit in a slightly different form and as part of a larger program—by a distinguished pioneer in stuttering therapy, Charles Van Riper (1973). I hope that the background provided in this chapter will encourage more clinicians and researchers to try the Lidcombe Program and to assess its effectiveness for the whole range of young children who stutter.

Brief History of Treatment of Stuttering in Young Children

Undoubtedly the first treatments for stuttering in children younger than 6 years were administered by parents. At some point in the evolution of speech and language, cave children began to stutter. Parents of some children probably corrected them and parents of others probably soothed them by speaking slowly. Results were undoubtedly mixed. Thus began the debate over how best to treat stuttering in early childhood.

The importance of this debate is related to what is at stake. There is ample evidence that, if treated early, as young children, individuals who stutter can recover normal speech; however, if treated late, as adolescents or adults, recovery is rarely complete (Starkweather, 1997). On the other hand, a large percentage of children who stutter recover without formal treatment (Yairi, 1999), and there is a concern among many parents and clinicians that early intervention that brings stuttering to children's attention may make recovery less likely (Silverman, 1988).

The recorded history of treatment of young children in the United States, Great Britain, Western Europe, and Australia, is the story of at least four different approaches. One is almost a century old (Froeschels, 1915). Parents and clinicians were warned not to call attention to their children's speech and especially not to their stuttering. The clinicians and researchers who advocated this approach treated preschool stuttering children only indirectly, working with parents to reduce communication pressures and life stresses on the children. Another approach was informal direct treatment administered by parents. Many parents, both on their own and with the advice of various professionals (e.g., Tomkins, 1916), told their children to stop stuttering and talk only when they could be fluent. A third approach, used by Van Riper and his disciples who worked directly with preschool children who stutter, rewarded fluency with positive and negative reinforcement, and had parents "restimulate" moments of stuttering with a fluent repetition of the stuttered word. They also worked with parents to make the child's environment more conducive to fluency. However, they, too, warned parents against calling attention to the child's stutters, using the rationale that "if he can be kept unaware of them [stutters], he will probably not develop the avoidance and struggle reactions which complicate the problem and are so difficult to extinguish" (Van Riper, 1973, p. 374). A fourth approach was more direct than Van Riper's, and built upon the systematic use of rewards or punishments shown to be effective with adults. Proponents included Ryan, Costello, and clinicians in Australia who developed the Lidcombe Program. In the following sections I describe these approaches and related constructs in more detail.

Indirect Approaches

As I have indicated, many early approaches to stuttering treatment of young children were indirect, admonishing parents not to correct the child's stuttering, nor even to call attention to it. In my own dog-eared copy of *First Aid for Stutterers,* Heltman (1943) gives this advice: "The first requirement is that parents cease worrying about it and stop calling it to his attention. His problem should not be discussed with his acquaintances and relatives, particularly in his presence" (p. 101).

This was the predominant approach in the 20th century for preschool children who stutter: to make their environments as facilitating to fluency as possible without calling attention to their stuttering. A Viennese physician, Emil Froeschels (1915), was a vocal champion of this view. He suggested that many children have effortless disfluencies when they begin to talk, but when parents or other listeners caution or correct them, children put unusual effort into their speech and develop real stuttering.

In much the same vein, Charles Bluemel, a British-born psychiatrist working in Denver, theorized that most children who stutter begin with very relaxed "primary stuttering" that they would normally outgrow (Bluemel, 1932). Unfortunately, according to Bluemel, many parents try to help them get over their stuttering by telling them to stop and start again without stuttering. This parental advice, Bluemel suggested, creates in the child anticipation of difficulty, struggle, and avoidance.

Diagnosogenic Theory of Stuttering Onset

Whereas most clinicians and researchers merely hypothesized that when children became aware of their disfluencies, they would then begin to struggle with them, Wendell

Johnson actually tested this hypothesis. The inspiration for this test was Johnson's passion for the field of general semantics, which promoted the belief that many problems are the result of the language people use in thinking and talking about them. Johnson theorized that stuttering was caused by people labeling a child's normal disfluencies as a problem that had to be fixed, thus creating a fear of disfluency in the child and subsequent hesitancy and struggle (Johnson et al., 1942). Under Johnson's guidance, a graduate student named Mary Tudor conducted a study of the effects of calling negative attention to the speech of normal speaking children (Tudor, 1939). Tudor screened the speech and language of all the children in an orphanage near the University of Iowa. She then selected 6 children (ages 5, 9, 11, 12, 12, and 15) who were normal speakers and told them that they were making errors in their speech and that they should try to speak more carefully. She also enlisted their caregivers to correct these children's speech when they made errors. Later, Tudor reassessed the children's speech and found that several of them had developed stuttering-like behaviors. Recent newspaper articles on the Tudor study (e.g., Dyer, 2001a, 2001b) have made it clear that, to produce these stuttering-like behaviors, extensive negative treatment was applied to these emotionally vulnerable children over several months and consisted not only of corrections and interruptions, but instructions as to how to speak and how to avoid stuttering.[1]

For several years prior to this study, Johnson and his colleagues began to study the disfluencies in normal children compared with those of children whose parents thought they were stuttering. Johnson's group found a great deal of overlap in the types of disfluencies reported by parents of both groups of children (Johnson et al., 1942). This evidence, coupled with the results of the Tudor study, led Johnson to develop the diagnosogenic theory of stuttering. This view suggested that the only cause of stuttering was parents' mislabeling of children's disfluencies as stuttering, and their corrections of these disfluencies. He later modified this extreme view to suggest that stuttering was caused by an interaction between the extent of the children's disfluencies, the listener's sensitivity to those disfluencies, and the children's sensitivity to their own disfluencies, and listeners' reactions (Johnson & Associates, 1959).

The views of Johnson, Froeschels, and Bluemel influenced a generation of speech–language pathologists, pediatricians, and journalists to warn parents never to call attention to their children's stuttering, and not to work directly on the child's speech. Instead, therapists worked indirectly, modifying children's environments to reduce stress and lower demands on speaking. In his book *The Treatment of Stuttering*, Van Riper (1973) summarized this popular belief, saying

> all of us wish to prevent the child from becoming aware of the interruptions in the flow of his speech. If he can be kept unaware of them, he will probably not develop the avoidance and struggle reactions which complicate the problem and are so difficult to extinguish. (p. 374)

In the 1980s the indirect approach was modified to include some more direct aspects, while keeping the focus on changing the child's environment. An example of this transitional view is given in the following section.

Capacities and Demands

Earlier beliefs that stuttering emerged solely as a result of parental correction of normal disfluencies gradually gave way to a broader concept of stuttering as the product of an

[1] After the writing of this chapter, a reanalysis of the Tudor data by Ambrose and Yairi (2002) showed that the experimental procedures produced no effects.

interaction between environmental pressures and factors within the child (Johnson & Associates, 1959). When evidence accumulated that many individuals who stuttered also showed deficits in the areas of language, articulation, and motor skill, researchers advanced hypotheses to relate these deficits to stuttering. Andrews and Harris (1964) and Neilson (1980) suggested that individuals who stutter have some neurological limitations in their capacities; their stuttering occurs when their capacities for fluency are stressed by demands related to speaking. This view was captured in the statement that "whether one will become a stutterer depends on one's neurological capacity . . . and the demand posed by the speech act" (Andrews et al., 1983). Starkweather further elaborated this view, suggesting that capacities include those for speech motor control, language development, social and emotional functioning, and cognitive ability. Demands include conversational, social, and emotional pressures from people in the child's environment and demands from within the child that may be made on all of these capacities (Starkweather, 1987, 1997; Starkweather, Gottwald, & Halfond, 1990).

The therapy for preschoolers that emerged from this model was aimed primarily at reducing the demands from the environment. However, some attention was given to increasing the child's and family's capacity for emotional resilience in response to the stuttering (Starkweather et al., 1990). Parent counseling and training, as well as direct and indirect therapy with the child, were incorporated into this approach. The family was educated about stuttering and taught that it is helpful to talk about stuttering with the child. Discussing stuttering openly with the child, commenting on moments of stuttering, and modeling an easy way of stuttering are all things that the family could do to help the child and themselves feel more comfortable with the child's speech. In this way they were reducing negative feelings that hinder recovery.

Considerable time was spent helping parents learn to make changes in the child's environment, particularly in verbal interactions. Parents were taught to use a speech rate and language level that were not too far above the child's level. They were encouraged to model easy disfluencies and comment on the child's speech rather than make negative nonverbal responses to his or her stuttering. They were shown how to develop turn-taking strategies for family conversations and spend daily one-on-one time with the child. They were helped to reduce verbal demands by commenting rather than questioning. And they were taught to do some of the direct therapy that the clinicians were doing with the child. Direct therapy activities included modeling and, if needed, stepwise reinforcement to teach easier and easier forms of stuttering. Some fluency shaping techniques such as gentle onset and light contacts were used. Starkweather et al. (1990) reported that 29 children who stuttered and their families completed the program and all children were speaking normally. The average duration of treatment was 12 sessions, but some took as many as 40 sessions. Most children required only 6 or 7 sessions.

Direct Approaches

Parent Correction of Stuttering Children

In the early part of the last century, some writers encouraged parents to correct their children. Tomkins (1916), in a journal article titled "Stammering and Its Extirpation," advised parents to refuse to listen to their children's stuttered speech and to tell them not to talk until they could be fluent. Despite the prevailing belief in the 1940s and 1950s that parents should never call attention to the child's stuttering, there is evidence that parental correction of their children's stuttering was often successful or at least did not impede spontaneous recovery. Glasner and Rosenthal (1957) found that more than 70% of parents they surveyed reported overtly correcting their children's stuttering and that many of the children who were reportedly corrected (48 out of 101) recovered. Those who advocated direct correction of stuttering children usually advised that it be done in a benign manner. For example, in a book of advice for parents of young children who stutter, Albright and Raaf suggested,

> Well meant advice such as "Stop and think about what you want to say," "Say that over more slowly," and "Take a deep breath before you speak" are excellent aids if they are spoken with calmness, tenderness, and friendliness on the part of the person giving advice. (Albright & Raaf, 1954, pp. 9–10, as cited in Van Riper, 1973)

The direct approach by parents, done in a nonsystematic manner, has never been carefully studied, and reports of positive outcomes must be viewed cautiously because so many children recover without formal treatment (Ingham, 1983).

Van Riper's Direct Approach

In his text on treating stuttering, Van Riper (1973) expressed impatience with the then-popular indirect approaches:

> The current belief so prevalent in this country [the United States] that no therapist should work directly with a child who has just begun to stutter is probably based on the equating of direct therapy with punishment. This is a mistake: it is possible to deal directly with the child's speech in many ways without hurting him or focussing on stuttering as an evil. (p. 385)

Van Riper went on to suggest that a clinician using his approach can work directly on fluency:

> He can make the child's speaking pleasant again;
>
> He can stimulate the child with models of fluency that are within the child's reach, models which, when imitated, will increase the child's own fluency;
>
> He can provide activities that integrate and facilitate the smooth flow of utterance;
>
> He can program schedules of rewards and reinforcements for fluency that will enhance it. (p. 399)

Describing his approach, Van Riper (1973) detailed how the clinician could give attention and appreciation to the child when the child spoke fluently, play games in which the child's fluent utterances are reinforced with food and prizes, and create activities in which the child had to produce a fluent utterance. The clinician or parent should respond to moments of severe stuttering by repeating what the child said, in a fluent way, without otherwise calling attention to it. In short, Van Riper advocated operant conditioning of fluency and stuttering and suggested that parents use it also, to increase fluency and decrease stuttering. It should be noted that this conditioning was done in a relatively nonsystematic way, that care was taken to avoid making the child highly aware of what was being reinforced, and that the operant conditioning was only a part of a larger therapy program that also included desensitization to stressors, and parent counseling to change the family environment.

Operant Conditioning

In the 1960s and 1970s, corrections and other punishments, as well as reinforcements and rewards, were used in more systematic ways as researchers began to develop a new approach to the treatment of stuttering: applied behavioral analysis. The harbinger of this approach was an article by Flanagan, Goldiamond, and Azrin (1958). Flanagan was a psychologist who had stuttered and had been treated successfully by Van Riper some years earlier. Goldiamond and Azrin were psychologists with experience in taking behavioral analysis out of the rat and pigeon laboratories and applying the principles and methods to human behavior. These experimenters demonstrated that negative reinforcement could be used to increase stuttering when escape from a loud noise was made contingent on moments of stuttering. They then showed that punishment could be used to decrease stuttering when the loud noise was made contingent on moments of stuttering. Extensive variations of this procedure were used for experimental treatment of adults who stuttered, particularly by researchers at Minnesota (e.g., Martin & Haroldson, 1969; Martin & Siegel, 1966).

Experimental operant conditioning with children who stutter was begun in the mid-1960s with the work of Rickard and Mundy (1965) and Leach (1969). Ryan (1971, 1974) developed programs for children as young as 6 years, which applied reinforcements to fluency and punishment to stuttering as they moved through hierarchies of more and more complex speaking situations, then transfer, and ultimately maintenance of fluency. Ryan's work with schoolchildren was particularly notable for its careful annotation of the use of programmed operant procedures to establish fluency and maintain it, and for its measurement of outcomes in real-world settings (Ryan & Van Kirk, 1974).

Despite the success of these experiments with adults and school-age children, there appear to be no published studies in the 1960s of reinforcement and punishment with preschool children who stuttered. Glasner and Rosenthal's (1957) report suggested, however, that many parents did successfully correct their stuttering children. Of the 101 preschool children who were reported to have received active correction by their parents (being told to slow down, repeat, stop and start over, and similar admonitions), only 36 were said to be still stuttering, whereas 48 had stopped stuttering and 17 were stuttering only occasionally. Van Riper (1973) had been using a treatment for preschool children that involved reinforcement for fluency. The time should have been ripe for studies of operant procedures for preschool children. However, the lay public as well as speech–language pathologists were still under the mandate not to call attention to a preschool child's stuttering. Johnson (1949) and Van Riper (1954, 1973) held strong positions, as indicated earlier, that children will outgrow their stuttering unless they become self-conscious of it. Johnson (1949) suggested that even too much praise for fluency can make a child self-conscious. Van Riper (1973) limited his concern to negative attention, which he thought would make the child struggle and avoid speaking in his efforts not to be disfluent.

A landmark study challenging this belief was conducted in the early 1970s by the same Minnesota researchers and clinicians who had studied operant procedures with adult and school-age stuttering children (see Chapter 2; see also Martin, Kuhl, & Haroldson, 1972). The study showed that stuttering reductions occurred and were shown to generalize to other situations and to be maintained at a 1-year follow-up evaluation. Thus it was shown that it is possible to call attention to stuttering in preschool children and thereby decrease its frequency. The more severely stuttering of the two children became so aware of the contingency that he said, "Hey, Suzybelle, how come you turn out when I'm stuttering, how come?"

Despite its radical nature, this study did not directly challenge the writings of Froeschels (1915), Bluemel (1932), or Johnson (1949), the progenitors of the indirect approach. These authors suggested that children with "primary" or effortless stuttering, and who are unaware of their stuttering should be managed in a way that does not make them self-conscious about their speech. The stuttering of the children in the Martin et al. (1972) study was severe enough that the children were aware of their stuttering. One subject "struggled (both audibly and nonaudibly) in excess of 15 seconds before saying a single word" (p. 745) and the other's stuttering at times "included marked tension in various muscles of the neck and face" (p. 748). Thus, before the experimental treatment, both had already developed the responses that Froeschels, Bluemel, and Johnson were afraid would result from negative attention to stuttering. A better test of this belief would be to use contingencies calling attention to stuttering with children whose disfluencies were multiple repetitions and prolongations without appreciable tension. This test awaited development of the Lidcombe Program, which applied contingencies to the effortless stutters of children who were apparently unaware of their stuttering prior to treatment.

Inspired by the work of Martin et al. (1972), Reed and Godden (1977) took the application of punishment one step further. The latter authors wanted to examine the effect of using the same type of verbal punishment employed by some parents of preschool children who stuttered. Authors such as Glasner and Rosenthal (1957) suggested that some parents had effectively treated their stuttering children by telling them to slow down. Reed and Godden used an ABA design to demonstrate that a preschool child's stuttering was reduced markedly when the experimenter told the child to slow down immediately after a moment of stuttering. During the extinction condition, when the experimenter stopped consequating stuttering, the child's stuttering returned to baseline levels. The experimenters then continued treatment with punishment for 15 more sessions and the child's stuttering decreased markedly. Recordings at home made during treatment and 8 months afterward showed stuttering to be reduced to 1% of words stuttered. The experimenters then treated another stuttering preschool child with the same punishment. Like the first child, this child reduced stuttering to very low levels and remained below 1% of words stuttered 8 months after treatment. Both these children had been stuttering with repetitions, prolongations, and facial tension prior to treatment.

In the early 1980s, Costello developed operant conditioning treatments for use with clients of all ages. Her approach paralleled that of Ryan (1971) and Ryan and Van Kirk (1974), but Costello explored operant treatments for preschool children as well. In a chapter on behavioral treatments for early childhood, Costello (1983) made a strong argument for the combined use of reinforcement and punishment with preschool children. She suggested (p. 83) that, in her clinical experience, children as young as 2 years can be treated successfully using tokens and praise (e.g., "That's really good talking!") for fluent utterances and verbal corrections for moments of stuttering (e.g., "Uh oh, I heard a bumpy word."). Costello designed her programs around gradual increases in the length of the child's utterances, controlled by the clinician, so that primarily fluent utterances occurred and punishment was infrequently needed. She reported that generalization often took place spontaneously, but that, when possible, she trained parents in the reinforcement component of the program and asked parents to carry out each step of the program at home, after it had been completed in the clinic, to help generalization. Costello indicated that she did not ask parents to correct the child's stuttering because she feared that parents might use punishment inappropriately.

At the same time as these operant clinicians were working directly on preschool children's stuttering, clinicians who favored less direct approaches were developing new ways of thinking about the relationships among children's stuttering, their abilities, and their environments.

What Is Traditional and What Is Different About the Lidcombe Program?

The preceding sections of this chapter have described both early and recent approaches to treating stuttering in preschool children. I now describe how the Lidcombe Program differs from those approaches as well as the ways in which it is similar.

Correcting and Calling Attention to Stuttering

In the 1980s and early 1990s, treatments for stuttering preschoolers were becoming more direct. A new generation of clinical scientists were experimenting with ways of talking with children about their stuttering without making them negatively self-conscious. Many were trying slow or "smooth" speech, along with reinforcement for fluency, and hierarchies of utterance length and complexity (Fosnot & Woodford, 1992; Pindzola, 1987). Others were working with children's natural speech, coupling reinforcement for fluency with punishment for stuttering (Costello, 1984). In the mid-1980s, Lidcombe clinicians and researchers began using operant procedures as the core treatment tool and tried out various components to see what would work best. After some initial failures, working largely with punishment for stuttering, the Lidcombe clinicians found that a combination of a large amount of reinforcement for fluency and a modicum of punishment[2] for stuttering worked best, especially when employed by parents. This combination, especially the corrections applied to stuttering, brought stuttering to the child's attention. Moreover, by using such speech-specific statements as "That was really smooth speech" and "Oops, that word was a little bumpy," parents enhanced the child's aware" clinicians typically discussed the child's stuttering with the parents while the child was present, treating the stuttering matter-of-factly, and thus reducing the potential for the child to become ashamed of it. Outcome studies (Lincoln & Onslow, 1997; Onslow, Andrews, & Lincoln, 1994) have demonstrated repeatedly that when young children are praised for fluency, corrected for stuttering, and otherwise made highly aware of their speech, their stuttering was reduced, not increased.

This evidence is at odds with what used to be "traditional" wisdom: that stuttering should not be brought to the young child's attention and that correcting a child's stuttering will make it worse. Traditional wisdom was probably based on cases observed by clinicians in which parents' nonsystematic corrections *did* make the child negatively self-aware and hesitant to speak. Indeed, Tudor's (1939) study provided some support for this hypothesis (see footnote 1). However, clinical procedures such as those of Costello (1983) and the Lidcombe Program appear to create a positive awareness of fluency and a relatively neutral awareness of stuttering in children. The reinforcement and punishment are systematic. And the children, unlike most of those in the Tudor (1939) study, are so young that their speech

[2]The word *punishment* is the formal operant word for a consequence that reduces the frequency of a behavior. However, *correction* will be used in its place because of the negative social connotations of the word punishment.

production systems may be highly malleable. These key differences may give children the capacity and motivation to work out for themselves what they need to do to become more fluent. Although I doubt most preschool children think like junior scientists, they may well work out intuitively and by trial and error what they have to do to be fluent. They may be helped along by the experience of mastery that results when they are fluent in the structured activities at the beginning of treatment and by the systematic praise they receive for their "good talking." Possibly most effective is the feedback they receive when they make mistakes, correct them, and receive more praise for their effectiveness at error correction.

Parents as Therapists

For generations, clinicians have invited parents of preschool children who stutter to become part of the therapy team. Parents' involvement has ranged from learning to change the child's environment (Gregory, 1999) to modeling easier stuttering at home (Starkweather et al., 1990) to consequating the child's stuttering with a fluent repetition of stuttered words (Van Riper, 1973). The Lidcombe Program has gone beyond having the parent as part of the therapy team and has pioneered the use of parents as the sole therapists for their children. (Sometimes both parents are involved in administering the therapy, but most often, in our experience, it is the mother alone who is the child's clinician.)

The use of the parent to deliver treatment in the Lidcombe Program has several advantages, but also some drawbacks. A major benefit is that the parents feel empowered. They are able to take action by working directly on the child's speech. Parents' anxieties appear to be reduced because, as a result of the daily and weekly data they collect, they see rapid changes in their child's fluency resulting from their efforts. Parents have also told me that they feel less guilty than they did when participating in other therapy programs. Their focus in the Lidcombe Program is on the child's speech rather than their own interaction patterns. Consequently, they are less worried that their own speech rates, interruptions, or complex vocabulary may have caused or worsened their child's stuttering.

Another major benefit is that parents learn to work independently when problems arise after the termination of formal therapy. This has been a characteristic of some other therapies, but not many. For example, one of our own experimental therapies had parents watch videotapes of their interactions with their child and decide for themselves what changes to make. This provided parents with the foundation for future work on their own (Guitar, Kopff-Schaefer, Donahue-Kilburg, & Bond, 1992). Gottwald and Starkweather's (1999) treatment prepares parents to treat their child's relapses on their own, by helping them to develop a plan for responding to future difficulties. In the Lidcombe Program parents are the primary clinicians for their children in structured conversations at home and in unstructured conversations from the beginning of treatment. Thus, they have become effective and confident in treating the child. Under the guidance of the speech–language pathologist, they learn to problem-solve as they tailor the program to their own children and negotiate bumps in the road to successful outcome.

Another advantage of having the parents deliver treatment has been noted by my colleague, Julie Reville. As service providers for their children, parents are diligently trained and counseled by the clinician, and will consequently feel they are the focus of the clinician's attention—more so than in child-centered approaches. This arrangement fosters parents' confidence and helps them become better able to meet their children's needs over the long term.

Among the drawbacks of the Lidcombe Program's parent-centered approach is that much depends on the willingness and ability of parents to deliver the treatment. Those families that are too busy or too distracted or have other limitations may not be able to meet the demands of this approach, which requires parents to conduct daily sessions with their child, rate the child's severity daily, and assess the child's stuttering frequency every week. A second problem that we have encountered is overzealous parents. Once given permission to praise and correct their children's speech, some parents go beyond guidelines for how frequently to reinforce fluency or correct stuttering. When we discover this, we are able to rein these parents in, but their children may take a little time to recover from too much of a good thing.

Daily Treatment in Structured Conversations with the Child

The Lidcombe Program requires that, in the first phase of treatment, the parent spends a little time every day in these one-on-one activities with the child. The parent and child engage in an activity that the child enjoys, and the parent praises the child's stutter-free speech. Praise flows freely because the activity is designed to elicit as much stutter-free speech as possible. This has the potential to give the child a sense of mastery in the skill of speaking. At the same time, the child's sense of security and well-being is probably enhanced by having a daily dose of parental undivided attention. Even as the treatment in structured conversations changes to include occasional corrections for stuttering, the one-on-one time and the frequent praise stay constant. As treatment in structured conversations is gradually replaced by treatment in unstructured conversations in a variety of new situations, the frequent praise is still on the daily menu. These elements may be particularly helpful for the temperamentally sensitive child, for whom stress may be a major mediator of stuttering.

Other therapies (e.g., Conture & Fraser, 1989; Guitar, 1998; Heinze & Johnson, 1985; Starkweather et al., 1990) also advocate one-on-one time every day. In most cases, the child is the focus of the parents' uninterrupted attention and is likely to feel that talking is fun. It is typically a situation in which the child is more fluent than usual and, in a general way, fluency is reinforced by the parents' attentive listening. If there is a difference in the Lidcombe Program's approach to this one-on-one time, it is the way the time is structured. Parents are taught how to elicit stutter-free speech and how to deliver immediate and contingent verbal stimulation. Moreover, the effectiveness of the parents' treatment in structured conversations is evaluated collaboratively at weekly meetings with the clinician, during which time the sessions are discussed, along with the parents' ratings of the child's speech.

Treatment in Unstructured Conversations

Many clinicians working with preschool stuttering (e.g., Prins, 1983) report spontaneous generalization of fluency from clinic or home sessions to daily talking situations. Some clinicians, such as Costello (1983), train parents to conduct program steps at home. However, the Lidcombe Program appears to be unique in training parents to use systematic procedures to obtain stutter-free speech in everyday speaking situations and to measure that achievement. It is not clear whether these procedures are necessary for stutter-free speech to occur in most everyday situations or to what extent it can generalize. As clinical researchers begin to "deconstruct" elements of the Lidcombe Program to study how and why it works, this information should become available.

Collection of Outcome Data and Speech Measures

Undoubtedly many experimental and clinical approaches to preschool children's stuttering have been effective. However, limited data are available on their real-world, long-term outcome. The exceptions appear to be the Stuttering Prevention and Early Intervention Approach used by Gottwald and Starkweather (1999; for outcomes see Starkweather et al., 1990, pp. 122–123) and the Lidcombe Program (e.g., Lincoln & Harrison, 1999). Both of these approaches show that early intervention can be both effective and efficient. However, the Lidcombe's Program training of parents to collect daily and weekly speech measures in all stages of treatment has the added benefit of giving parents and clinicians more detailed information. This means that the elements of treatment, such as praise and correction, can be fine-tuned regularly to meet each child's needs, not only during Stage 1 of treatment but for the long term as well. It also provides parents with clear evidence of their children's improvement, increasing their confidence in their ability to provide treatment.

Conclusion

This chapter has attempted to show the historical context in which the Lidcombe Program was developed and its relationship to other current clinical approaches to early stuttering. Although the Lidcombe Program draws on many sources, it has many unique elements. Among the most important, in my judgment, are (a) the use of parents as primary service deliverers, (b) the use of systematic verbal reinforcement and corrections delivered by parents, (c) the frequency of treatment in structured conversations by parents, (d) the systematic delivery of verbal contingencies in the unstructured conversations of real-life speaking situations, (e) the open discussion of stuttering with and around the child, and (f) the feedback available from regular measures of the child's stuttering so that the clinician can help the parent determine immediately if treatment recommendations have been successful. Why and how the Lidcombe Program works and which of its components are critical to success are questions yet to be answered.

Although one motivation for writing this chapter was to encourage clinicians to learn and then try the Lidcombe Program, another was to encourage research on the components of the treatment and on comparisons of the program with other approaches and with spontaneous recovery. There are many new areas to explore and a wealth of clinical studies to be conducted.

In summary, the Lidcombe Program has a respectable pedigree. Its more controversial aspects, which have raised some resistance to its acceptance, may be among its most effective components. Its eventual impact will be determined not on how well it can be integrated into current theories and practices, but on whether it makes a significant, long-lasting, and beneficial change in the communication skills of preschool children who stutter. The prospects look good.

Acknowledgments

This chapter is dedicated to Julie Reville and Melissa Bruce, two superb clinicians at the University of Vermont who have pioneered the use of the Lidcombe Program in the

United States. They have been my mentors as I have learned to work with preschool children using the Lidcombe Program. I would like to acknowledge my good fortune of being taught the Lidcombe Program by Rosalee Shenker and JoAnne Wilding at the Montreal Fluency Centre. Finally, I would like to thank my colleagues Rebecca McCauley, Melissa Bruce, and Julie Reville for their helpful editorial comments on this chapter.

References

Ambrose, N. G., & Yairi, E. (2002). The Tudor study: Data and ethics. *American Journal of Speech–Language Pathology, 11*, 190–223.

Andrews, G., Craig, A., Feyer, A.-M., Hoddinott, S., Howie, P., & Neilson, M. (1983). Stuttering: A review of research findings and theories circa 1982. *Journal of Speech and Hearing Disorders, 48*, 226–246.

Andrews, G., & Harris, M. A. (1964). *The syndrome of stuttering*. London: Willam Heinemann.

Bluemel, C. (1932). Primary and secondary stammering. *Quarterly Journal of Speech, 18*, 187–200.

Conture, E., & Fraser, J. (1989). *Stuttering and your child: Questions and answers*. Memphis, TN: Speech Foundation of America.

Costello, J. (1983). Current behavioral treatments for children. In D. Prins & R. Ingham (Eds.), *Treatment of stuttering in early childhood: Methods and issues* (pp. 69–112). San Diego: College-Hill Press.

Costello, J. M. (1984). Treatment of the young chronic stutterer: Managing fluency. In R. F. Curlee & W. H. Perkins (Eds.), *Nature and treatment of stuttering: New directions* (pp. 375–395). San Diego: College-Hill Press.

Dyer, J. (2001a, June 10). Ethics and orphans: The "monster study." *San Jose Mercury News* (CA), p. 1a. Retrieved June 30, 2001, from http://www.mercurycenter.com

Dyer, J. (2001b, June 11). An experiment leaves a lifetime of anguish. *San Jose Mercury News* (CA), p. 1a. Retrieved June 30, 2001, from http://www.mercurycenter.com

Flanagan, B., Goldiamond, I., & Azrin, N. (1958). Operant stuttering: The control of stuttering behavior through response-contingent consequences. *Journal of the Experimental Analysis of Behavior, 1*, 173–177.

Fosnot, S. M., & Woodford, L. L. (1992). *The fluency development system for young children*. Buffalo, NY: United Educational Services.

Froeschels, E. (1915). The significance of symptomatology for understanding of the essence of stuttering. *Folia Phoniatrica, 4*, 217–230.

Glasner, P., & Rosenthal, D. (1957). Parental diagnosis of stuttering in young children. *Journal of Speech and Hearing Disorders, 22*, 288–295.

Gottwald, S., & Starkweather, C. W. (1999). Stuttering prevention and early intervention: A multiprocess approach. In M. Onslow & A. Packman (Eds.), *The handbook of early stuttering intervention* (pp. 53–82). San Diego: Singular Publishing Group.

Gregory, H. (1999). Developmental intervention: Differential strategies. In M. Onslow & A. Packman (Eds.), *The handbook of early stuttering intervention* (pp. 83–101). San Diego: Singular Publishing Group.

Guitar, B. (1998). *Stuttering: An integrated approach to its nature and treatment* (2nd ed.). Baltimore: Williams & Wilkins.

Guitar, B., Kopff-Schaefer, H., Donahue-Kilburg, G., & Bond, L. (1992). Parent verbal interaction and speech rate. *Journal of Speech and Hearing Research, 35*, 742–754.

Heinze, B., & Johnson, K. (1985). *Easy does it: Fluency activities for young children*. East Moline, IL: LinguiSystems.

Heltman, H. J. (1943). *First aid for stutterers*. Boston: Expression Company.

Ingham, R. J. (1983). Spontaneous remission of stuttering: When will the emperor realize he has no clothes on? In D. Prins & R. J. Ingham (Eds.), *Treatment of stuttering in early childhood: Methods and issues* (pp. 113–135). San Diego: College-Hill Press.

Johnson, W., et al. (1942). A study of the onset and development of stuttering. *Journal of Speech Disorders, 7*, 251–257.

Johnson, W. (1949). An open letter to the mother of a stuttering child. *Journal of Speech and Hearing Disorders, 14*, 3–8.

Johnson, W., & Associates. (1959). *The onset of stuttering*. Minneapolis, MN: University of Minneapolis Press.

Leach, E. (1969). Stuttering: Clinical application of response-contingent procedures. In B. B. Gray & G. England (Eds.), *Stuttering and conditioning therapies* (pp. 115–127). Monterey, CA: Monterey Institute for Speech and Hearing.

Lincoln, M., & Harrison, E. (1999). The Lidcombe Program. In M. Onslow & A. Packman (Eds.), *The handbook of early stuttering intervention* (pp. 103–117). San Diego: Singular Publishing Group.

Lincoln, M., & Onslow, M. (1997). Long-term outcome of an early intervention for stuttering. *American Journal of Speech–Language Pathology, 6*, 51–58.

Martin, R., & Haroldson, S. (1969). The effects of two treatment procedures on stuttering. *Journal of Communication Disorders, 2*, 115–125.

Martin, R., Kuhl, P., & Haroldson, S. (1972). An experimental treatment with two preschool stuttering children. *Journal of Speech and Hearing Research, 15*, 743–752.

Martin, R., & Siegel, G. (1966). The effects of simultaneously punishing stuttering and rewarding fluency. *Journal of Speech and Hearing Research, 9*, 466–475.

Neilson, M. (1980). *Stuttering and the control of speech: A systems analysis approach*. Unpublished doctoral dissertation, University of New South Wales, Kensington, Australia.

Onslow, M., Andrews, C., & Lincoln, M. (1994). A control/experimental trial of an operant treatment for early stuttering. *Journal of Speech and Hearing Research, 37*, 1244–1259.

Pindzola, R. H. (1987). *Stuttering intervention program: Age 3 to grade 3*. Austin, TX: PRO-ED.

Prins, D. (1983). Continuity, fragmentation, and tension: Hypotheses applied to evaluation and intervention with preschool disfluent children. In D. Prins & R. Ingham (Eds.), *Treatment of stuttering in early childhood: Methods and issues* (pp. 21–42). San Diego: College-Hill Press.

Reed, C., & Godden, A. (1977). An experimental treatment using verbal punishment with two preschooler stutterers. *Journal of Fluency Disorders, 2*, 225–233.

Rickard, H. C., & Mundy, M. B. (1965). Direct manipulation of stuttering behavior: An experimental-clinical approach. In L. P. Ullman & L. Krasner (Eds.), *Case studies in behavior modification* (pp. 268–274). New York: Holt, Rinehart & Winston.

Ryan, B. P. (1971). Operant procedures applied to stuttering therapy for children. *Journal of Speech and Hearing Disorders, 36*, 264–280.

Ryan, B. P. (1974). *Programmed therapy of stuttering in children and adults*. Springfield, IL: Charles C Thomas.

Ryan, B. P., & Van Kirk, B. (1974). The establishment, transfer, and maintenance of fluent speech in 50 stutterers using delayed auditory feedback and operant procedures. *Journal of Speech and Hearing Research, 39*, 3–10.

Silverman, F. (1988). The "monster" study. *Journal of Fluency Disorders, 13*, 225–231.

Starkweather, C. W. (1987). *Fluency and stuttering*. Englewood Cliffs, NJ: Prentice Hall.

Starkweather, C. W. (1997). Therapy for younger children. In R. Curlee & G. Siegel (Eds.), *Nature and treatment of stuttering: New directions* (pp. 257–279). Boston: Allyn & Bacon.

Starkweather, C. W., Gottwald, S. R., & Halfond, M. H. (1990). *Stuttering prevention: A clinical method*. Englewood Cliffs, NJ: Prentice Hall.

Tomkins, E. (1916). Stammering and its extirpation. *Pedagogical Seminary, 23*, 151–174.

Tudor, M. (1939). *An experimental study of the effects of evaluative labeling on speech fluency*. Unpublished master's thesis, University of Iowa, Iowa City.

Van Riper, C. (1954). *Speech correction: Principles and methods* (3rd ed.). Englewood Cliffs, NJ: Prentice Hall.

Van Riper, C. (1973). *The treatment of stuttering*. Englewood Cliffs, NJ: Prentice Hall.

Yairi, E. (1999). Spontaneous recovery and clinical trials research in early childhood stuttering: A response to Onslow and Packman (1999). *Journal of Speech, Language, and Hearing Research, 42*, 398–409.

Chapter 4

The Timing of Early Intervention with the Lidcombe Program

Ann Packman, Mark Onslow, and Joseph Attanasio

There is now consensus in the literature dealing with early stuttering that it is desirable to intervene in the first few years after onset. Consequently, there are many treatments available for such intervention (see Onslow & Packman, 1999a). However, there is no such consensus in the literature about *when* to intervene, the main reason being that many preschool children recover from stuttering without treatment.

There is some debate about the terminology surrounding recovery from stuttering without treatment, concerning whether it should be known as spontaneous recovery or natural recovery (see Finn, 1997). Our preference is for the latter, as it implies that the recovery is influenced by natural forces in the child's life, whether innate or environmental. Environmental factors possibly influencing natural recovery would include, for example, advice given to children by parents such as "Slow down," "Start again," and so on (for a review see R. J. Ingham, 1983). As we see it, this type of informal intervention contrasts with the systematic procedures included as part of a professional intervention such as the Lidcombe Program.

Until as recently as 1984 (see Andrews, 1984), it was argued that treatment for early stuttering should be delayed until it is clear that the child is unlikely to recover naturally. This position reflects the "wait-and-hope" approach: In other words, "Let's wait and hope that the stuttering goes away naturally. If it doesn't, then we will treat." At first glance, the wait-and-hope approach has some appeal. It can be argued that treating children who are destined to recover anyway is a waste of clinical resources and an unnecessary burden on families. However, a number of other factors need to be considered if treatment is delayed, including whether leaving a child to stutter for a number of years will have adverse effects, even though the child eventually recovers, and whether responsiveness to treatment is compromised if the child is still stuttering after a wait-and-hope period has elapsed.

Fortunately, considerably more evidence exists now than in 1984 to inform decisions about when to treat stuttering in young children. Indeed, this issue has recently been the subject of lively debate (see Bernstein Ratner, 1997; Curlee & Yairi, 1997, 1998; R. J. Ingham & Cordes, 1998; Packman & Onslow, 1998, 1999; Zebrowski, 1997). Although a number of writers advocate treating stuttering in the first year or two after onset, it appears that there is still considerable reluctance to do so, at least in the United States (Bernstein Ratner, 1997). Interestingly, this is not necessarily the case in other countries. In Australia, for example, the development of the Lidcombe Program prompted suggestions that children be treated as soon as possible after the onset of stuttering (Onslow, 1996), and ideally within the first 6 months (Packman & Lincoln, 1996).

The purpose of this chapter is to develop guidelines for intervention with the Lidcombe Program. We do not think that the guidelines we present will necessarily apply to other treatments. An analysis of stuttering treatments for children (R. J. Ingham & Cordes, 1998) suggested that treatment is more likely to be effective if introduced within 15 months of onset. However, our research indicates that this is not necessarily the case with the Lidcombe Program (Jones, Onslow, Harrison, & Packman, 2000).

There is now considerably more information about the Lidcombe Program than there was when Packman and Lincoln (1996) speculated about the timing of early intervention. We also now know much more about natural recovery from stuttering than we did at that time. These two ever-increasing bodies of knowledge provide the basis for the development in this chapter of guidelines for the timing of early intervention with the Lidcombe Program. When deciding when to intervene, the clinician will want to consider what is known about natural recovery, such as rate and predictors of recovery, and balance this against what is known about recovery with the Lidcombe Program, such as whether certain factors influence responsiveness to treatment.

The clinician will also need to consider other factors relating to the individual child and family; factors for which evidence is inconclusive or nonexistent. For example, as yet there is no evidence to inform us about when to implement the Lidcombe Program with a child who stutters and also has another form of communication disorder. The circumstances of the individual family are also relevant when planning intervention. Thus, decisions about when to treat will be guided by evidence but will also take into account clinician judgment. As we see it, there is no one decision that will apply to every child.

This chapter explores the options for a clinician who has decided that a preschool child is stuttering and that the treatment of choice is the Lidcombe Program. The chapter overviews research findings that are relevant to the timing of early intervention with the Lidcombe Program and then suggests guidelines for the decision-making process, drawing on the available evidence and consideration of other factors. The findings relevant to the decision-making process are (a) rate of natural recovery, (b) time to natural recovery, (c) predictors of natural recovery, (d) effectiveness of the Lidcombe Program, (e) treatment time required for recovery with the Lidcombe Program, (f) predictors of treatment time required for recovery with the Lidcombe Program, (g) the psychological impact of stuttering on children, and (h) the psychological impact of stuttering on families.

Research Findings

Rate of Natural Recovery

It has been known for many years that some children who begin to stutter will recover without formal treatment. Many of the earlier writings on this topic relied on prevalence data. It has been known for some time that the prevalence of stuttering in children is around 5% and in adults only around 1% (Bloodstein, 1995). The logical conclusion from this, then, is that many children—perhaps around 80%—recover naturally (Curlee & Yairi, 1997). Such estimates, however, have not been without controversy (see R. J. Ingham & Cordes, 1998).

The first report of prospective data on the onset and course of stuttering came from a 1,000-family study in England conducted from 1946 to 1962 (see Andrews & Harris, 1964; see Box 4.1 for an overview of the study). The findings of that study indicated that around 78% of children who started stut-

Box 4.1

More than 1,000 children born in Newcastle-upon-Tyne in May and June of 1947 were followed up to age 15 years, although some dropped out of the study. The children were checked regularly by health workers and seen by a speech therapist if speech and language development was thought to be delayed. Of the 43 children who reportedly started to stutter, 30 did so before the age of 6, the age that is relevant to the present discussion. Of those, stuttering persisted (at least to age 15) in 7 children, and 23 (78%) recovered. Of those who recovered, 16 (70%) apparently recovered within about 6 months, two (7%) recovered within a year, and the rest took longer than a year, with one child recovering after stuttering for about 10 years. It should be noted that some of the children in the study apparently had treatment for their stuttering (Andrews, 1984).

tering in the preschool years subsequently recovered, a finding that supported previous estimates.

At the time of writing, a large prospective epidemiological study, the Illinois Early Childhood Stuttering Project, is under way in the United States (for a description of the project, see Yairi & Ambrose, 1999; see also Box 4.2 for an overview of the project). Estimates of natural recovery from this project are similar to previous estimates, ranging at the present time from 75% to 89% (see Packman & Onslow, 1998). A recent report of 84 children who were followed for at least 4 years since the onset of stuttering (Yairi & Ambrose, 1999) indicated that 74% of them recovered naturally. The authors suggest, however, that this is an underestimation, because children with brief bouts of stuttering would probably not have been included in the project.

Another longitudinal study of 1,021 preschool children conducted in Denmark (Mansson, 2000; see Box 4.3 for an overview of the study) suggests a recovery rate of 85%.

Although estimates of natural recovery vary, the longitudinal studies referred to indicate a recovery rate of around 80%. However, it is important to note that treatment may be a confounding variable in such longitudinal studies, regardless of the ultimate recovery

Box 4.2

At the time of writing, the Illinois Early Childhood Stuttering Project is in progress. Yairi and colleagues are recruiting from the community children who have started stuttering within the previous 12 months. The project aims to establish the epidemiology of early stuttering, including rate of recovery and predictors of recovery (e.g., see Ambrose, Cox, & Yairi, 1997; Paden, Yairi, & Ambrose, 1999; Watkins & Yairi, 1997; Watkins, Yairi, & Ambrose, 1999; Yairi & Ambrose, 1999; Yairi, Ambrose, Paden, & Throneburg, 1996). Children are assessed for a number of factors, such as number and type of stuttering-like dysfluencies, phonological and linguistic development, and family history of stuttering. They are reassessed at regular intervals and, over time, are deemed as either recovered or persistent.

Box 4.3

Mansson (2000) reported a longitudinal study of all children who were born on an isolated island county of Denmark during 1990 and 1991. This resulted in 1,021 children being followed to age 9 years. The first speech–language evaluation occurred around the children's 3rd birthday, and the children were reevaluated 2 years and 4 years later. Of these children, 51 were reported to have started to stutter by age 3 years and another 2 children were reported to have started stuttering after that. At the second assessment (at around age 5 years) 71% no longer stuttered, whereas at the third assessment (at around age 9 years) 85% no longer stuttered. The treatment history of the children is unclear.

status of the children. This confound appears to be unavoidable, given the ethical problems of withholding treatment from young children for a number of years. By the same token, natural recovery may be a possible confounding variable in treatment research (Packman & Onslow, 1998).

When applying recovery data to the clinical context, it is important to remember that the longitudinal studies reported recruited subjects from the general population rather than from speech clinics. Consequently, recovery rates for children whose parents bring them to the speech clinic because of stuttering are likely to be much lower. Parents do not typically bring their children to the clinic immediately following onset, and may not become concerned until the child has been stuttering for some months, or even years. Thus many children who experience short periods of stuttering will never present to a speech clinic. It would be incautious, then, for clinicians to generalize the recovery rate of around 80% to their clinical caseload (Packman & Onslow, 1998). It is not possible to provide general information on the recovery rate in the clinical population, as this would vary depending on clinics, communities, cultures, attitudes to stuttering, access to clinical services, and media-driven awareness of available treatments. In any event, recovery in a clinical population is likely to be considerably less than the 80% (or thereabouts) reported in epidemiological studies.

Time to Natural Recovery

Although the clinician is interested in knowing how many children recover naturally, the time taken to natural recovery is also relevant. This information would allow an informed decision about when a child would no longer be likely to recover without treatment.

The Newcastle upon Tyne study is informative on this issue (see Box 4.1). Although the raw data for the children in that study are not available, recovery times can be estimated from the figures (e.g., see Figure 1.1 in Andrews, 1984). As discussed in Box 4.1, 70% of preschoolers in this study apparently recovered within about 6 months, another 7% recovered within 1 year, and the rest (23%) took longer than a year, with one child recovering after about 10 years. Again, caution is required in considering these data in the clinical context. Many of the children in that data set who appeared to have a transient bout of stuttering lasting less than 6 months would be unlikely to present to a clinic. The Illinois Project also provides information on the time it takes for children to recover naturally. In a report of 84 children participating in the project, Yairi and Ambrose (1999) state that "duration of stuttering tends to run from 6 to 35 months for most, with some children stuttering as long as 3 to 4 years before recovery" (p. 1104). The Mansson (2000) report indicates that onset in almost all children occurred before age 3 years, and of these children 71% had recovered within 2 years. Recovery occurred for the other children some time later. A report of a single case (J. C. Ingham & Riley, 1998) showed natural recovery occurring, without any treatment, over more than 3 years.

It is difficult to make a general statement about time to recovery, based on these findings. Also, the information that is available needs to be interpreted cautiously, in terms of its relevance to the clinical context. Clearly, however, recovery can occur many years after onset. The best we can conclude from the available evidence is that many children recover within 1 year of onset, but that a child who has been stuttering for 2 years or longer may still recover naturally.

Predictors of Natural Recovery

Knowing whether certain factors predict natural recovery would inform the decision-making process, and establishing this information is one of the aims of the Illinois Project. Results of this project to date indicate that phonological and language skills may influence whether a child recovers naturally, but that their role in recovery is far from clear (Yairi & Ambrose, 1999). Results from the project also suggest that family history of natural recovery may be associated with natural recovery. However, the only factors that can be considered to predict natural recovery are being a girl and being close to onset. It is well known that many more girls than boys recover naturally and that the longer a child has been stuttering the greater the odds that child will not recover. One important finding from the Illinois Project that is relevant here is that stuttering severity does not predict natural recovery. In other words, a child whose stuttering is severe is as likely to recover naturally as a child whose stuttering is mild.

Although some evidence suggests that certain factors tend to be associated with natural recovery, it is not possible to say whether a particular child will or will not recover on the basis of those factors. Thus, although the actuarial data (described previously) tell us what percentage of children in a group are likely to recover naturally, and even the characteristics those children tend to possess, those data tell us nothing about the prospects of natural recovery for an individual child. It is important to remember that the clinician cannot say that even a child for whom the odds are favorable—for example, a girl who has been stuttering for only a couple of months—will recover naturally (see Bernstein Ratner, 1997).

Effectiveness of the Lidcombe Program

The clinician will want to take the effectiveness of the Lidcombe Program into account when considering when to intervene. Most important, the clinician will want to know whether the program is more effective than letting nature run its course. In other words, if the program is implemented, will it have an impact on the natural course of stuttering?

Outcome studies have shown that stuttering rate reduces to zero, or near zero, after intervention with the Lidcombe Program (Onslow, Andrews, & Lincoln, 1994; Onslow, Costa, & Rue, 1990) and that after treatment children's speech is likely to be indistinguishable from that of control children (Lincoln, Onslow, & Reed, 1997). However, it is still not known, definitively, whether those outcomes can be attributed to the treatment. In other words, treatment effectiveness has not yet been demonstrated. There are two related issues to consider here (see Packman

& Onslow, 1998): (1) whether the program will eliminate stuttering in a child who will not recover naturally and (2) whether the program has an immediate ameliorative effect on stuttering, regardless of whether the child is destined to recover naturally.

As far as the first issue is concerned, as discussed above, it is not possible to know in advance whether a child is going to recover naturally. The only way to address the issue, then, is to show that stuttering reduces to a greater extent in a group of children who receive treatment than in a similar group who do not. This would indicate that treatment had an effect on stuttering that was over and above that of natural recovery. Such a study would involve withholding treatment for many years, to ensure that all children in the control group who were destined to recover naturally did so. As discussed above, this is ethically unacceptable. However, a [randomized controlled trial currently under way in New Zealand (see Jones, Gebski, Onslow, & Packman, 2001; see also Chapter 14) will contribute to establishing the efficacy of the Lidcombe Program. In this trial the control group receives any treatment that would normally be offered, provided it is not the Lidcombe Program.

Until the results of this trial are available, however, there are at least two reasons to believe that the Lidcombe Program is more effective than natural recovery (see Onslow & Packman, 2001). First, data show that stuttering reduces to very low levels in school-age children who participate in the program (Lincoln, Onslow, Lewis, & Wilson, 1996). In other words, Lincoln et al. showed that the program is still effective with children in the 7- to 12-year-old group who are unlikely to recover naturally. Second, the factors that predict responsiveness to the Lidcombe Program (discussed later) are different from those that predict natural recovery (discussed previously). For example, children with mild stuttering take less time to recover with the Lidcombe Program than children whose stuttering is more severe. However, stuttering severity does not predict natural recovery. Taken together, these findings strongly suggest that there is a treatment agent in the Lidcombe Program that is independent of natural recovery.

The second efficacy issue is whether the Lidcombe Program positively affects the natural course of stuttering, regardless of whether natural recovery might occur at some time in the future. This is an important issue, and the clinician needs to be confident that implementing the program will have an immediate impact on stuttering. This was shown to be the case in a recent study by Harris, Onslow, Packman, Harrison, and Menzies (in press). Ten preschool-age children who received the Lidcombe Program had significantly lower stuttering rates after 12 weeks than a nontreated control group of children measured over the same period. This preliminary study demonstrated the immediate impact of the program on stuttering, without the need to withhold treatment for a long period.

In summary, then, outcome data are available for the Lidcombe Program, but we still await efficacy data. However, clinicians can have considerable confidence that the Lidcombe Program, should it be implemented, will have an ameliorative effect on stuttering, whether or not the child is destined to recover naturally at some future time.

Treatment Time Required for Recovery with the Lidcombe Program

The treatment time needed for recovery with a program is important because the clinician needs to know how long to set aside for treatment. The clinician may also want to balance the possible benefits of early implementation of a program against the demands the program places on the family. Take the example of a child who is moderately distressed about stuttering. The clinician may feel that immediate intervention with the Lidcombe Program is warranted to alleviate the distress. However, as the distress is not severe, the clinician may also consider delaying intervention for some period. Treatment is time consuming, so the clinician may judge it preferable to wait a little longer to see if the child recovers naturally.

The available evidence suggests that, for most children, Stage 1 of the Lidcombe Program does not take an overly long time. Jones et al. (2000) provided recovery plots for treatment with the Lidcombe Program, indicating how long preschool-age children took to complete Stage 1 (see Boxes 1.7 and 4.4 for overviews of this study). The median treatment time was 11 weekly clinic visits, with the 90th percentile at 22 visits. Allowing for occasional missed visits, that brings median treatment time in at around 3 months. We know, then, that 50% of children will take less than 3 months to complete Stage 1 and 50% will require more than 3 months, with 90% of children completing Stage 1 within 6 months.

Predictors of Treatment Time Required for Recovery with the Lidcombe Program

In deciding when to intervene, clinicians will want to know whether there are any factors that predict responsiveness to treatment. Time since onset of stuttering is of particular interest. For example, clinicians will want to know whether delaying intervention (increasing onset-to-treatment time) means that a child will take longer to benefit from the program. If this is true, most clinicians would probably decide to implement treatment as soon as possible after onset. If responsiveness is not related to the time since onset, however, delaying treatment would be an option. This is probably the most important issue to consider—although not the only one—in

Box 4.4

A file audit of 250 preschool children who had completed Stage 1 of the Lidcombe Program at The University of Sydney and at the Stuttering Unit, Bankstown Health Service (Jones, Onslow, Harrison, & Packman, 2000), gathered information from clinic files on the time taken to complete Stage 1 of the program, age, gender, time since onset, and stuttering severity. The median number of weekly clinic visits taken to complete Stage 1 was 11, which confirmed previous findings (Onslow, Andrews, & Lincoln, 1994), and 86% of children had completed Stage 1 within 20 clinic visits. Logistic regression indicated that children with more severe stuttering took longer to complete Stage 1 than children with less severe stuttering. However, neither increasing age nor onset-to-treatment time were associated with longer treatment time. In other words, delaying treatment for a period after onset of stuttering apparently does not jeopardize responsiveness to treatment with the Lidcombe Program. The children in this study were all younger than 6 years, ranging from 27 to 71 months of age. Thus, the findings of this study relate only to children in the preschool-age group and cannot be generalized to older children.

deciding when to intervene with the Lidcombe Program.

The results of Jones et al. (2000) indicated that delaying treatment for a short period after onset does not increase the time taken to complete Stage 1 of the program. In fact, the findings suggested that children who had been stuttering longer took slightly less time to complete Stage 1. This may be a function of age and associated cognitive development, rather than time since onset per se. This idea is supported by reports from clinicians that older children respond to the program in a way that suggests they become involved at a cognitive level. For example, they are more likely to say, "I didn't have any bumpy words!" than are younger children. The Jones et al. findings also showed that children whose stuttering tended to be more severe took longer to complete Stage 1 than children whose stuttering was less severe.

When taking account of the results of Jones et al. (2000) in deciding when to implement the Lidcombe Program, it is important to remember that the children in that study were all of preschool age; that is, they were younger than 6 years. Thus, the results of the study cannot be generalized to older children. Indeed, there is evidence to indicate that delaying intervention with the Lidcombe Program past the preschool years may jeopardize responsiveness to treatment. The results of Lincoln et al. (1996) suggest that, although school-age children also respond to the program, they are likely to take longer to complete Stage 1 and are probably more likely to fail to meet program criteria at some time during Stage 2.

A prospective study currently under way is investigating other factors that might predict treatment recovery time. Predictor factors in this study include linguistic and phonological development. It will be helpful to know, for example, if children with delayed language take longer to complete Stage 1 than children with normal or superior language development.

The Psychological Effects of Stuttering on Children

If a clinician is contemplating delaying treatment for some period, the psychological effects of stuttering on the child need to be considered. If a child is distressed by the stuttering, then this would seem to be an important factor in the decision-making process.

Yairi (1983) reported that, of 22 parents of young stuttering children, 23% said that their child was aware of stuttering when it first began, and 18% said that their child was distressed by stuttering when it first began. In a survey of parents of preschool children who stutter (Onslow, Harrison, & Jones, 1993), 30% of the 121 respondents reported that their child was aware of their stuttering and was reacting negatively to it, in many instances immediately after onset. The following are some of the verbal and nonverbal reactions of children to their own stuttering, as reported by parents in the Onslow et al. study:

> At first he attempted to yell, sing or whisper the word to make it come out and became so frustrated he would cover his mouth with his hand, tea towel—anything just to stop it.

> One night while lying quietly in bed he told me—without a stutter—that he was having trouble talking, sometimes.

> Within a few days of the stuttering starting, he was saying "Mummy I can't talk properly."

> She would put her hand to her mouth, and she would get angry with herself and sometimes hit her mouth with her hand and say "I can't say it."

> He was asking for a drink and got stuck on the words "can," "I," "a" and before finishing slumped to the floor, cried and said he couldn't talk any more.

> He kept hitting his mouth as if his mouth was being naughty and required a smack and this was pathetic to watch. Two relatives were in

tears when they saw this frustration he had when trying to speak.

Interestingly, too, it seems that nonstuttering children as young as 3 years identify stuttering, and at 4 years of age children may evaluate stuttering negatively (Ezrati-Vinacour, Platzky, & Yairi, 2001). There is also evidence that preschool children who stutter may be teased by their peers (see Chapter 20; see also Onslow et al., 1993). Parental reports on teasing in the Onslow et al. (1993) survey included the following:

> She was unable to communicate fluently—was embarrassed at preschool—other children teased her.
>
> Embarrassment and teasing at prekindergarten class.
>
> Other children were making fun of him. And he asked me, "Mummy why do I talk funny?"

Such reports of child frustration and alarm, and of teasing by other children, could be considered grounds for implementing treatment immediately. It can certainly be argued that implementing the program would lead to a reduction of the distress in these children in a quite short period.

Not all preschool children appear distressed or psychologically disturbed by their stuttering, however. A preliminary study using contemporary psychological instruments showed no behavioral or emotional disturbances in 8 stuttering preschool children (Woods, Shearsby, Onslow, & Burnham, 2002; see Box 4.5 for an overview of this study). Furthermore, it is not known whether children who are frustrated by their stuttering, or teased because of it, will suffer any long-term psychological problems if treatment is delayed for some period within the preschool years. In summary, the effects of distress and teasing on the psychological well-being of the young stuttering child, in the short term and over a number of years, are not clear. Nonetheless, clinicians may judge, in light of individual circumstances, that a child's distress is sufficient grounds for implementing the program.

The Psychological Effect of Stuttering on Families

As far as we are aware, no research has been directed specifically at the psychological effects of early stuttering on families. However, the findings of the Woods et al. (2002) study, which aimed to detect any deterioration in child behavior and child–parent relationships as a result of the Lidcombe Program, are relevant to this topic. In this

Box 4.5

Woods, Shearsby, Onslow, and Burnham (2002) investigated psychological variables in 8 preschool-age children before starting the Lidcombe Program and after completing Stage 1. Instruments were the *Child Behaviour Checklist* (CBCL; Achenbach, 1988, 1991) and the *Attachment Q-set* (AQS; Waters, 1995). The CBCL is completed by the parent and detects child anxiety, aggression, withdrawal, and depression. The AQS is also completed by the parent and measures the degree of attachment between mother and child. All children scored within normal limits on these two measures before treatment, and there were no clinically significant changes in the measures after treatment.

study, the 8 preschool-age children and their mothers scored normally on the assessment procedures both before and after the treatment. In other words, there was no evidence from this study that stuttering had negatively affected the child–parent relationships.

Nonetheless, parents and other family members are frequently distressed by stuttering in their preschool child, and concern for the child's welfare is usually what prompts parents to bring the child to the speech clinic anyway. Parents often report feelings of guilt, believing they have done something to cause the child to start stuttering. This is not surprising, given that the onset of stuttering typically occurs after a period of apparently normal speech development. Another scenario is that concern and guilt are common where one parent also stutters. The parent may feel responsible for genetically transmitting stuttering to the child. Also, the parent whose own stuttering has caused negative life consequences may feel apprehensive for the child and request immediate intervention.

Again, these feelings may be seen as grounds for arguing that the program should be implemented immediately. However, the long-term effects of family distress are not known and, in any event, other options for easing family distress, such as counseling, should be considered before implementing treatment. Nonetheless, clinician judgment is important here, and in some cases the clinician may decide that implementing the program immediately is in the best interests of the family.

The Decision-Making Process

When a parent brings a child to the speech clinic and it is confirmed that the child is stuttering, the clinician needs to decide when to implement the Lidcombe Program. Is the presence of stuttering sufficient grounds for implementing the program immediately, or should implementation of the program be delayed for some period, to see if natural recovery occurs? And if implementation is delayed, for how long should it be delayed?

Consider the Evidence

We have presented the available evidence on a number of issues that bear on the decision-making process. Many of the findings are meager and preliminary; nonetheless, they provide at least some evidence on which to base the decision in question. Of course, this decision would be straightforward if we could know in advance whether a particular child will recover naturally. Treatment could then be reserved for those who will not recover. Unfortunately, at present we do not have that luxury. We can estimate the odds for recovery for an individual child by looking at factors associated with recovery, such as gender and time since onset, but beyond those factors we cannot tell whether an individual child will or will not recover naturally.

What can we say, then, taking into account the available evidence, about when to implement the Lidcombe Program? We make three general statements that we suggest form the basis for the decision-making process. First, without taking any other factors into account, it is thought preferable to allow a child to recover naturally than to place the considerable demands of the program on the child and family. Second, it is not possible to predict whether an individual child will or will not recover naturally. Third, delaying the implementation of the Lidcombe Program for some period *within the preschool years* does not appear to reduce a child's responsiveness to it.

Together, these statements suggest that delaying treatment to see if natural recovery occurs is the clinician's first option. The caveat to this is that treatment should be implemented by age 6 years. Evidence for the Lidcombe Program is derived primarily from children younger than 6 years of age, and there is reason to believe that implementation of the program at some time after this age may jeopardize the child's responsiveness to it.

Other Factors

Although the consideration of evidence is important for accountable decision making, there are other factors that need to be considered but for which little or no evidence is available and about which no general statements can be made. Such factors include the psychological effects of stuttering on the child and the family (as discussed previously), the presence of a concomitant communication disorder, and individual family circumstances. In the clinician's judgment, consideration of these factors may suggest overriding a decision to delay treatment.

Concerning the psychological effects of stuttering on the child, the decision whether to intervene immediately because a child is distressed will depend on the individual child. How distressed is the child? For how long has the child been distressed? Is the child's anguish distressing the family? Is the child sufficiently distressed to justify implementing the Lidcombe Program immediately? Each case will be different and the answer to these questions will be different for each child. When taking this factor into account, the decision when to intervene will be guided by the judgment of the clinician concerned. As far as the psychological effects of stuttering on the family are concerned, we have found in almost all cases where a family is distressed by their child's stuttering that they are reassured when informed that (a) their child may recover naturally, (b) there are excellent outcome data for the Lidcombe Program, and (c) delaying the program within the preschool years is unlikely to jeopardize the child's responsiveness to it. If the family is not reassured by this information, then further counseling may be required. Although it does not seem to us that family distress alone is sufficient grounds for implementing the Lidcombe Program, there is no evidence one way or the other. Again, clinicians will consider each case individually and make the decision judged to be appropriate for the individual family.

The second consideration is the presence of another communication disorder. Children who come to a speech clinic because of stuttering frequently have another communication disorder, such as delayed speech or language, and the issue of which disorder to treat first, or whether to treat the disorders simultaneously, has been addressed extensively in the general stuttering literature (see Guitar, 1998, for an overview).

There is no evidence to indicate that any one approach is superior when implementing the Lidcombe Program with such children. Stuttering is likely to complicate therapy for another disorder, such as language delay, because children who stutter may reduce grammatical complexity in an attempt to reduce their stuttering. Thus, the presence of stuttering may mean that the child will not benefit maximally from that therapy. The same would hold for therapy for a phonological disorder, where children may curtail their verbal output, and perhaps avoid saying certain words, in an attempt to minimize their stuttering. It could be argued, then, that it is preferable to treat stuttering first, so that the child can benefit more from therapy for the other disorder. If the child is already having treatment for the coexisting disorder, this treatment could be suspended and reintroduced after the child completes Stage 1 of the Lidcombe Program. This would be, then, after a median of 11 weekly sessions—not an unduly long time to suspend the other treatment. Stuttering can then be kept under environmental control by the clinician, if necessary, with the occasional verbal contingency such as "smooth talking" or "that was a bit bumpy." However, there is no evidence to support this position, and the clinician may in fact decide to delay implementing the Lidcombe Program for some period, if this is judged to be in the best interests of the child. In short, the clinician will consider the circumstances relating to each child in deciding what course of action to take.

Finally, many other individual circumstances relating to the family may influence the decision about when to implement the program. Family members fall ill sometimes, families relocate, babies are born, and parents stop and start work. A circumstance that is commonly considered is when a child is due to start "big school" in a few months. Some parents request that treatment be implemented before the child starts school because of the logistical constraints on clinic attendance that going to school can entail.

To summarize, the clinician can embark on the decision-making process with some confidence that it is unlikely that the child's responsiveness to the Lidcombe Program will be jeopardized by waiting for some period after onset, as long as the program is implemented within the preschool years. However, that guideline may be overridden and treatment implemented earlier if the clinician decides that doing so is warranted. In short, the clinician decides whether it is preferable, on balance, to implement the Lidcombe Program immediately or to delay implementation for some period.

We are not suggesting that delaying the implementation of the Lidcombe Program means that no further action is required. On the contrary, once consulted by a family, the clinician has a duty of care. In effect, delaying treatment can be seen as an intervention strategy in itself (see Onslow & Packman, 1999b) and should incorporate frequent monitoring, as suggested by R. J. Ingham and Cordes (1998). This process is also similar to that proposed by Onslow (1992) for managing children for whom stuttering status is unclear. The Monitoring Program we advocate involves systematic checking by the clinician for trends in stuttering rate and severity, and for signs of the onset of—or an increase in—distress in the child or family.

We have found that an effective way to monitor stuttering is to teach parents how to use the 10-point severity scale used in the Lidcombe Program (see Chapter 5) so that they can record their child's stuttering severity each day. The parent makes phone or e-mail contact with the clinician at regular intervals and reports the severity of the child's stuttering for each day.[1] In addition, the child and parent visit the clinic at regular intervals, perhaps every month, so that the clinician can measure stuttering rate (see Chapter 5) and check for child and family distress. The trends in stuttering measures can be taken into account when deciding when to implement the program with a child who is in the Monitoring Program. For example, at some point during the Monitoring Program a child may start to show clear signs of distress about stuttering, yet at the same time the stuttering measures may indicate that stuttering is improving. Rather than implement the program at that point, the clinician may deide to wait a little longer to see if the child recovers naturally.

In any event, the program is implemented if at any time during the monitoring process the clinician judges that, in light of other factors, this is warranted. If the child recovers naturally while on the Monitoring Program, the frequency of monitoring is re-

[1] At present we are designing a monitoring procedure whereby parents dial a telephone number and record daily severity ratings using their telephone keyboard. Software analysis of these data assists the clinician to detect any systematic temporal trends in the severity ratings.

duced but monitoring continues for up to a year, so that any recurrence of stuttering does not go undetected. The Lidcombe Program should be implemented for any remaining children before they reach 6 years of age.

The guidelines for deciding when to intervene with the Lidcombe Program that we have suggested are shown in Figure 4.1. When a preschool child first comes to the speech clinic and the child is identified as stuttering, the clinician has two options. Option 1 is to delay implementing the Lidcombe Program for some period, and Option 2 is to implement the program as soon as practicable. Option 1 should be considered first; however, Option 2 is available if the clinician judges that certain factors (as discussed previously) warrant it (e.g., if the child is approaching age 6 or if the child is very distressed). In the latter case, the Lidcombe Program is implemented as soon as practicable. If the clinician selects Option 1, the child enters the Monitoring Program. The child continues in the Monitoring Program and the Lidcombe Program is implemented if at any time the clinician decides this is warranted. If the child does not recover naturally while in the Monitoring Program, the Lidcombe Program is implemented before the child reaches 6 years of age.

Conclusion

The guidelines for deciding when to intervene with the Lidcombe Program that are proposed in this chapter are based on the evidence available at the time of writing. As we stated earlier, however, much of this evidence is preliminary and in need of replication with greater numbers of subjects. At present, research findings about the epidemiology, nature, and treatment of early stuttering are proliferating rapidly, so it is likely that the evidence guiding decisions about the timing of intervention will change over the next few years.

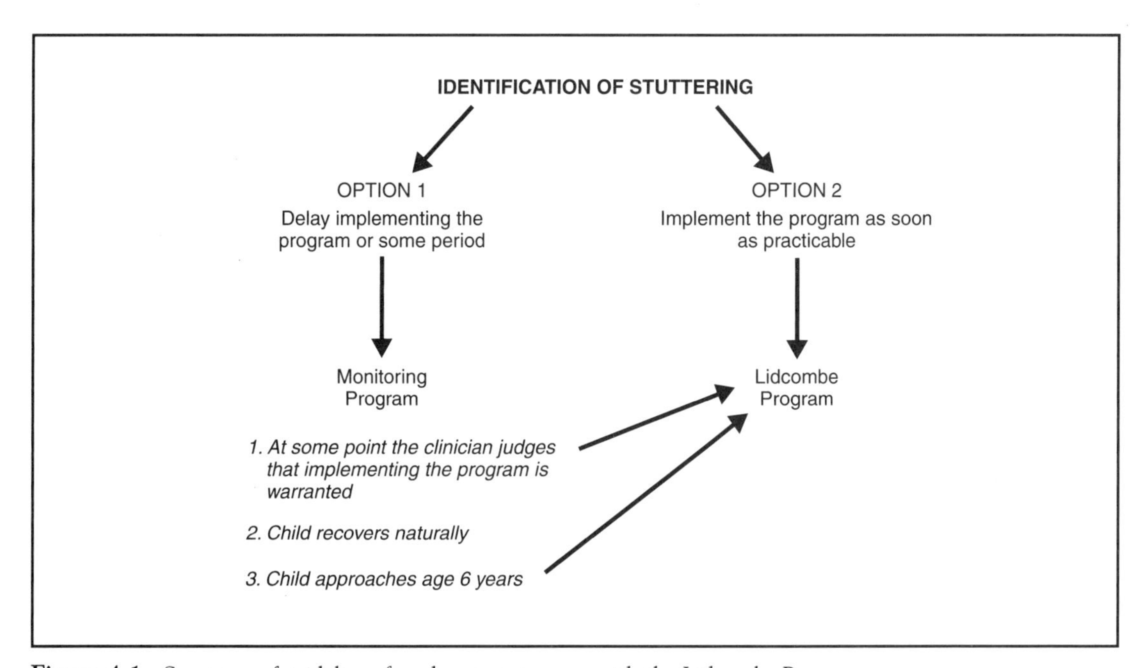

Figure 4.1. Summary of guidelines for when to intervene with the Lidcombe Program.

References

Achenbach, T. M. (1988). *Child behavior checklist for ages 2–3*. Burlington: University of Vermont.

Achenbach, T. M. (1991). *Manual for the child behavior checklist/4–8 and 1991 profile*. Burlington: Department of Psychiatry, University of Vermont.

Ambrose, N. G., Cox, N. J., & Yairi, E. (1997). The genetic basis of persistence and recovery in stuttering. *Journal of Speech, Language, and Hearing Research, 40*, 567–580.

Andrews, G. (1984). The epidemiology of stuttering. In R. F. Curlee & W. H. Perkins (Eds.), *Nature and treatment of stuttering: New directions* (pp. 1–12). Philadelphia: Taylor & Francis.

Andrews, G., & Harris, M. (1964). *The syndrome of stuttering*. London: William Heineman.

Bernstein Ratner, N. (1997). Leaving Las Vegas: Clinical odds and individual outcomes. *American Journal of Speech–Language Pathology, 6*, 29–33.

Bloodstein, O. (1995). *The handbook of stuttering* (5th ed.). San Diego: Singular Publishing Group.

Curlee, R., & Yairi, E. (1997). Early intervention with early childhood stuttering: A critical examination of the data. *American Journal of Speech–Language Pathology, 6*, 8–18.

Curlee, R., & Yairi, E. (1998). Treatment of early stuttering: Advances and research needs. *American Journal of Speech–Language Pathology, 7*, 20–26.

Ezrati-Vinacour, R., Platzky, R., & Yairi, E. (2001). The young child's awareness of stuttering-like disfluency. *Journal of Speech, Language, and Hearing Research, 44*, 368–380.

Finn, P. (1997). Adults recovered from stuttering without formal treatment: Perceptual assessment of speech normalcy. *Journal of Speech, Language, and Hearing Research, 40*, 821–831

Guitar, B. (1998). *Stuttering: An integrated approach to its nature and treatment* (2nd ed.). Baltimore: Williams & Wilkins.

Harris, V., Onslow, M., Packman, A., Harrison, E., & Menzies, R. (in press). An experimental investigation of the impact of the Lidcombe Program. *Journal of Fluency Disorders*.

Ingham, J. C., & Riley, G. (1998). Guidelines for documentation of treatment efficacy for young children who stutter. *Journal of Speech, Language and Hearing Research, 41*, 753–770.

Ingham, R. J. (1983). Spontaneous remission of stuttering: When will the emperor realize he has no clothes on? In D. Prins & R. J. Ingham (Eds.), *Treatment of stuttering in early childhood: Methods and issues* (pp. 113–135). San Diego: College-Hill Press.

Ingham, R. J., & Cordes, A. (1998). Treatment decisions for young children who stutter: Further concerns and complexities. *American Journal of Speech–Language Pathology, 7*, 10–19.

Jones, M., Gebski, V., Onslow, M., & Packman, A. (2001). Design of randomized controlled trials: Principles and methods applied to a treatment for early stuttering. *Journal of Fluency Disorders, 26*, 247–267.

Jones, M., Onslow, M., Harrison, E., & Packman, A. (2000). Treating stuttering in young children: Predicting treatment time in the Lidcombe Program. *Journal of Speech, Language, and Hearing Research, 43*, 1440–1450.

Lincoln, M., Onslow, M., Wilson, L., & Lewis, C. (1996). A clinical trial of an operant treatment for school-age children who stutter. *American Journal of Speech–Language Pathology, 5*, 73–85.

Lincoln, M., Onslow, M., & Reed, V. (1997). Social validity of an early intervention for stuttering: The Lidcombe Program. *American Journal of Speech–Language Pathology, 6*, 77–84.

Mansson, H. (2000). Childhood stuttering: Incidence and development. *Journal of Fluency Disorders, 25*, 47–57.

Onslow, M. (1992). Identification of early stuttering: Issues and suggested strategies. *American Journal of Speech–Language Pathology, 1*, 21–27.

Onslow, M. (1996). *Behavioral management of stuttering*. San Diego: Singular Publishing Group.

Onslow, M., Andrews, C., & Lincoln, M. (1994). A control/experimental trial of an operant treatment for early stuttering. *Journal of Speech and Hearing Research, 37*, 1244–1259.

Onslow, M., Costa, L., & Rue, S. (1990). Direct early intervention with stuttering: Some preliminary data. *Journal of Speech and Hearing Disorders, 55*, 405–416.

Onslow, M., Harrison, E., & Jones, A. (1993, May). *Early stuttering: Onset, treatment and recovery*. Paper presented at the annual conference of the Australian Association of Speech and Hearing, Darwin.

Onslow, M., & Packman, A. (Eds.). (1999a). *Handbook of early stuttering intervention*. San Diego: Singular Publishing Group.

Onslow, M., & Packman, A. (1999b). The Lidcombe Program and natural recovery: Potential choices of initial management strategies for early stuttering. *Advances in Speech Language Pathology, 1*, 113–121.

Onslow, M., & Packman, A. (2001). The Lidcombe Program of early stuttering intervention: Awaiting the results of a randomised controlled trial. *Asia-Pacific Journal of Speech, Language, and Hearing*, 6, 85–89.

Packman, A., & Lincoln, M. (1996). Early stuttering and the Vmodel. *Australian Journal of Human Communication Disorders*, 24, 45–54.

Packman, A., & Onslow, M. (1998). What is the take-home message from Curlee and Yairi? *American Journal of Speech–Language Pathology*, 7, 5–9.

Packman, A., & Onslow, M. (1999). Recovery from early stuttering: Clarifying some issues. *American Journal of Speech–Language Pathology*, 8, 94–95.

Paden, E. P., Yairi, E., & Ambrose, N. C. (1999). Early childhood stuttering: II. Initial status of phonological abilities. *Journal of Speech, Language, and Hearing Research*, 42, 1113–1124.

Waters, E. (1995). Appendix A: The Attachment Q-Set (version 3.0). In E. Waters, B. E. Vaugh, G. Porsada, & K. Komdo-Ikemura (Eds.), Caregiving, cultural, and cognitive perspectives and secure-base behavior and working models: New growing points of attachment theory and research. *Monographs of the Society for Research in Child Development*, 60 (Serial No. 244), pp. 234–246.

Watkins, R. V., & Yairi, E. (1997). Language production abilities of children whose stuttering persisted or recovered. *Journal of Speech, Language, and Hearing Research*, 40, 385–399.

Watkins, R. V., Yairi, E., & Ambrose, N. G. (1999). Early childhood stuttering: III. Initial status of expressive language abilities. *Journal of Speech, Language, and Hearing Research*, 42, 1125–1135.

Woods, S., Shearsby, J., Onslow, M., & Burnham, D. (2002). Psychological impact of the Lidcombe Program of early stuttering intervention: Eight case studies. *International Journal of Language and Communication Disorders*, 37, 31–40.

Yairi, E. (1983). The onset of stuttering in two- and three-year-old children: A preliminary report. *Journal of Speech and Hearing Disorders*, 48, 171–177.

Yairi, E., & Ambrose, N. G. (1999). Early childhood stuttering: I. Persistency and recovery rates. *Journal of Speech, Language, and Hearing Research*, 42, 1097–1112.

Yairi, E., Ambrose, N., Paden, E. P., & Throneburg, R. N. (1996). Predictive factors of persistence and recovery: Pathways of childhood stuttering. *Journal of Communication Disorders*, 29, 51–77.

Zebrowski, P. (1997). Assisting young children who stutter and their families: Defining the role of the speech–language pathologist. *American Journal of Speech–Language Pathology*, 6, 19–28.

Part II

Procedures

Chapter 5

Measuring Stuttering

Michelle Lincoln and Ann Packman

Stuttering has been measured by clinicians and researchers since at least the 1930s (Bloodstein, 1995). In the clinical setting, measuring stuttering enables the clinician to quantify the extent of the problem and also to ascertain the effect of treatment. With the current emphasis on accountability and evidence-based practice in speech–language pathology, it is becoming increasingly important that clinicians show that their interventions have a positive effect on impairment, which, in this case, is the behaviors of stuttering. Stuttering measures are also important in clinical research, particularly in establishing the outcomes and efficacy of various treatments.

Although there is general agreement on the need to measure stuttering in the clinic and in research, there is no consensus in the current literature about how this should be done, or even what behaviors should be counted (see Packman & Onslow, 1998). The choice of stuttering measures in the Lidcombe Program is guided by the fact that the treatment is behavioral, and that stuttering and stutter-free speech are the primary behavioral responses. Thus, stuttering, rather than disfluency, is measured in the program. Three measures of stuttering are used in the Lidcombe Program. Two of these are behavioral, namely rate and frequency of stuttering, and one is nonbehavioral, namely judgments of stuttering severity. General features of these measures are discussed briefly, and the rest of the chapter outlines the implementation and role of the measures in the Lidcombe Program.

Stuttering Measures

Stuttering Rate

The measure of stuttering rate used in the Lidcombe Program is percentage of syllables stuttered (%SS). The %SS is calculated from the number of syllables spoken and the number of those syllables that were unambiguously associated with stuttering. The use of a button-press counting device reduces the demands of this counting task, which means the clinician can use the device to measure stuttering in real time, that is, while the child is speaking or while an audiotape recording of the child speaking is playing. To use the device, the clinician presses one button for every syllable that is judged to be free of stuttering and an adjacent button for every syllable that is judged to be stuttered. The total syllables spoken is the sum of the two. The device automatically calculates and displays total syllables and %SS. Measuring %SS on-line in this manner requires training.

We emphasize at this point that the %SS measure relies on perceptual judgments of stuttering, because the listener makes a judgment about whether each syllable is or is not stuttered. This is different from behavioral counts of disfluencies used by other investigators in the current literature, such as Stuttering-Like Disfluency (SLD; Yairi & Ambrose, 1999). Box 5.1 provides a discussion of the differences between SLDs and %SS.

Because the %SS measure rests on judgments about whether or not syllables are stuttered, the reliability of the measure needs to be established. To do this, in research at least, another listener is typically recruited to independently measure %SS for the same speech samples. The reliability (agreement between listeners) of measures of stuttering rate has been questioned (see Ingham & Cordes, 1992). However, outcome studies of the Lidcombe Program suggest that the reliability of %SS measures does not appear to be a problem when measuring the stuttering rate of young children (see Box 5.2).

Stuttering Severity

Measuring stuttering severity involves assigning a score on a scale where the highest score indicates *extremely severe stuttering* and the lowest score represents *no stuttering*. These Likert-type scales are used widely in speech–language pathology and they have a number of advantages for measuring stuttering. First, they give an indication of overall severity, not merely a rate of stuttering as is the case with the %SS measure. Second, they are easy to use, requiring little training. Third, they are intuitive, in that most people are familiar with the idea of giving something a score out of, say, 10. This makes the scales suitable for use by parents, as occurs in the Lidcombe Program. Fourth, they do not require that the child produce a sample of speech in a certain time frame, as the %SS measure does. A severity rating can refer to stuttering severity over a considerable period, during which the child may speak infrequently or sporadically. Fifth, the procedure requires no instruments. The final advantage, which is related to the fifth, is that the covert nature of the procedure means that the child is unaware of it, thus eliminating reactivity to assessment. In turn, this makes this type of rating particularly suitable for obtaining a valid measure of stuttering rate in naturalistic speaking situations.

Likert-type scales usually have 5 or 7 points. However, a 10-point scale was developed for use in the Lidcombe Program (see Onslow, Andrews, & Costa, 1990) to make it more user-friendly for parents. It was thought that parents would be more comfortable assigning a score out of 10, rather than out of 5 or 7. The findings of Onslow, Andrews, et al. (1990) showed that parents can use a 10-point scale reliably to track variations in stut-

Box 5.1

To obtain a measure of Stuttering-Like Disfluencies (SLDs), a listener counts the following disfluency types: (a) single-syllable word repetition, (b) part-word repetition, and (c) disrhythmic phonation (for a discussion of the confusion surrounding this term, see Packman & Onslow, 1998). Because these definitions do not distinguish between stuttered and nonstuttered disfluencies, SLD is not a measure of stuttering per se (see Wingate, 2001). Thus, although 3 SLDs per 100 syllables is typically used to delineate stuttering and nonstuttering children, a child who displays 1 SLD per 100 words may still be stuttering. In contrast, percentage of syllables stuttered (%SS) is a measure of the rate of unambiguous stuttering. Thus, a child who displays 1%SS would be considered to be stuttering.

Box 5.2

Interjudge agreement (reliability) of percentage of syllables stuttered (%SS) measures is reported in a number of outcome studies of the Lidcombe Program (Lincoln & Onslow, 1997; Lincoln, Onslow, Lewis, & Wilson, 1996; Onslow, Andrews, & Lincoln, 1994).

Onslow et al. (1994) established the reliability of %SS measures for 12 preschool-age children who completed the Lidcombe Program. The measures were made from audiotape recordings of the children speaking in everyday situations, before and after treatment. The measures were made blind by a clinician who was experienced in measuring stuttering but who was independent of the study. Percentage of syllables stuttered measures were made blind on 36 of these recordings (six from each child) by another clinician who again was independent of the study. Agreement between the two clinicians was clearly high for most subjects, although there was some discrepancy between the scores in some subjects. In all but one child, both sets of %SS scores indicated that stuttering dropped to very low levels after treatment.

Interjudge agreement for %SS outcome measures of the 11 school-age children studied by Lincoln et al. (1996) was assessed by having an independent judge perform %SS measures on two 30-minute audiotape recordings of each child speaking in his or her natural environment, one made before treatment and one made after treatment. As reported by Lincoln et al., for some children there were considerable differences in the %SS measures between the original and the independent judges. However, in all cases the independent judge confirmed that stuttering severity decreased markedly after treatment and that, with the exception of one child, stuttering remained around or below 1%SS after treatment.

Similarly, in the long-term outcome study reported by Lincoln and Onslow (1997), interjudge and intrajudge agreements for %SS measures after treatment were assessed with 30 and 96 comparisons, respectively. Each of these data points was a 10-minute speech sample. For interjudge agreement, 91% of the comparisons differed by less than 1%SS, and for intrajudge agreement, 93% of the comparisons differed by less than 1%SS.

tering severity in everyday speaking situations (see Box 5.3).

Stuttering Frequency

Stuttering frequency is a measure of how often stuttering occurs in a given period, namely, stutters per minute of speaking time (SMST). The time the child spends talking is measured with a cumulative stopwatch, and the number of stutters that occur during that period is recorded, usually with pen and paper. The number of stutters is divided by the child's talking time to calculate SMST.

Implementing Stuttering Measures

Percentage of Syllables Stuttered

In the Lidcombe Program, the clinician typically measures %SS at the start of each clinic visit. To this end, the clinician, parent, or

Box 5.3

In Onslow, Andrews, and Costa's (1990) study, four parents audiotaped their children speaking in everyday situations on four occasions each day, for 6 days. Each parent then listened to the recordings of his or her own child and assigned each speech sample a score from 1 to 10. They repeated the task 1 to 2 months later. An experienced clinician listened to all the recordings and also assigned severity scores, and a second experienced clinician listened to all the recordings and counted the number of stutters. Three of the parents were highly consistent in their use of the severity scale from the first to the second occasion, and their scores agreed to a satisfactory extent with those of the clinician. The fourth parent did not use the scale reliably, showing low consistency and agreement. The severity scores of this parent, however, correlated quite highly with the stutter counts of the second clinician. All four parents used the range of scores provided by the scale to track changes in severity in their children. The authors concluded that a 10-point scale of stuttering severity has reliability, validity, and utility. They cautioned, however, that parents may need training in use of the scale.

both engage the child in naturalistic conversation usually during a play activity, and the clinician uses the counting–timing device described previously to measure %SS while the child is speaking. This can usually be done unobtrusively. However, if the child is distracted by the procedure, compliance may be increased by having the child press the buttons and look at the display for a short while. To be valid, the %SS measure should be based on a sample of at least 300 syllables.

The clinician enters the %SS score graphically on the child's data sheet, which the clinician keeps in the file. An example of the data sheet designed for use with the Lidcombe Program is shown in Figure 5.1. It shows the stuttering measures for Stage 1 of the program for a preschool child, William. The left vertical axis is %SS and the right vertical axis is severity, as measured by the severity rating scale. The horizontal axis is time, in days. The open circles show William's %SS scores, which were made once a week at the clinic visit. At the first clinic visit, William's stuttering rate was high, at 18%SS. His %SS scores varied considerably over the first 4 weeks, but by Week 5 a downward trend in %SS was apparent. At Week 10, William was no longer stuttering in the clinic and 0%SS was recorded through to Week 15.

Sometimes children are reluctant to talk in the clinic. This means that the clinician hears very little speech from the child. If the child is simply shy when talking to the clinician, the problem can usually be solved by the clinician's opting out of the conversation on which the %SS measure is based and leaving the parent to help generate a speech sample from the child. However, the child may still provide very limited amounts of speech in the clinic, and the %SS measure may be considered invalid. In this case, measures of the rate of stuttering can be obtained from recordings of the child speaking in everyday situations. Fortunately, the scenario where the clinician is unable to obtain any valid within-clinic %SS measure is rare.

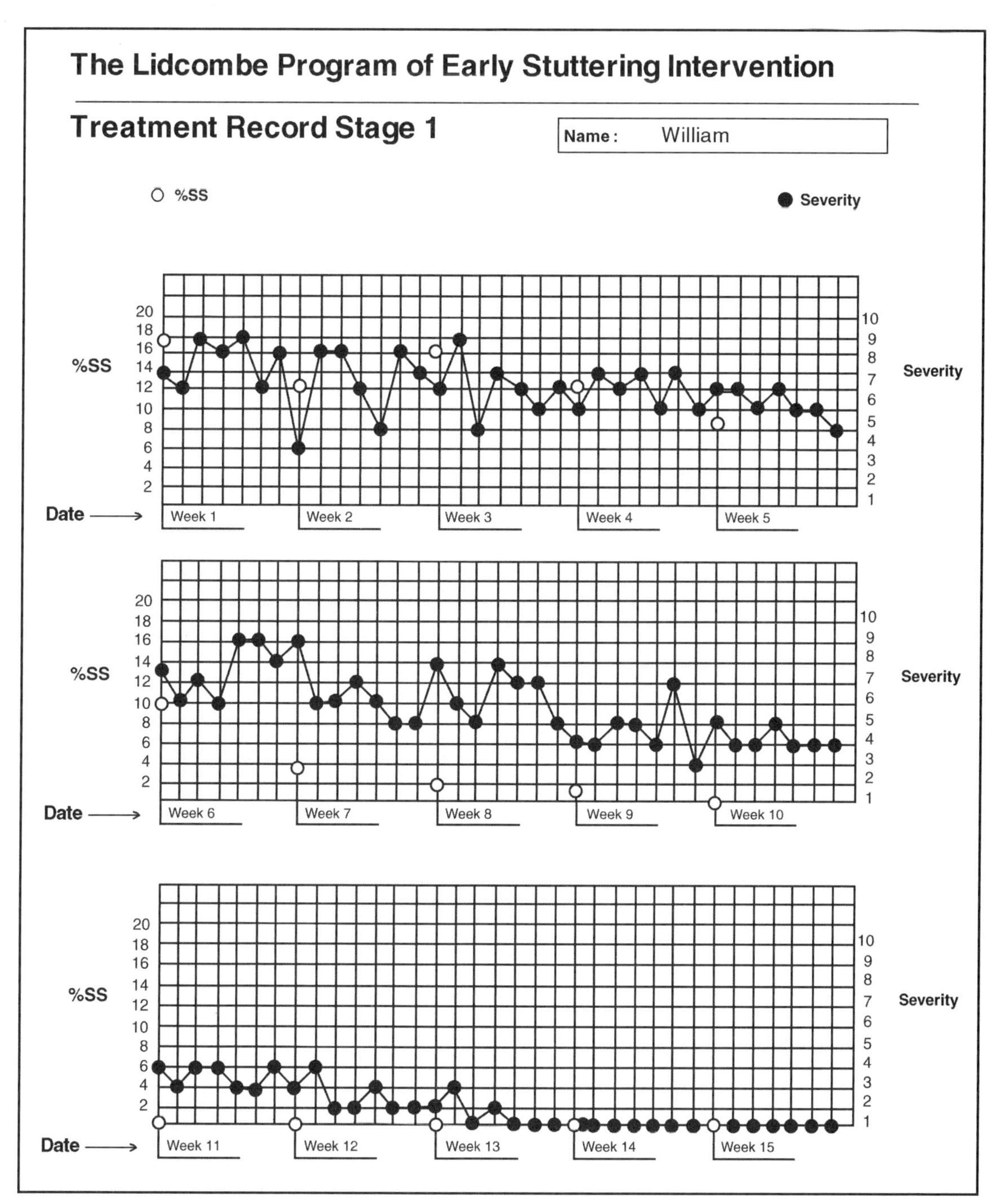

Figure 5.1. Example of data sheet used in the Lidcombe Program to record percentage of syllables stuttered (%SS) and stuttering severity.

Severity Ratings

In the Lidcombe Program, the parent rates the severity of the child's stuttering each day, based on the speech the child produces in naturalistic situations. A 10-point rating scale is used, where 1 = *no stuttering*, 2 = *very mild stuttering*, and 10 = *extremely severe stuttering*. This is a slightly modified version of the scale developed by Onslow, Andrews, et al. (1990). The clinician trains the parent in the use of the scale as soon as the program begins. The clinician describes the scale to the parent and then asks the parent to assign a severity rating (SR) from 1 to 10 to the speech sample on which the clinician made the %SS measure at the start of the clinic visit. The clinician suggests to the parent that a score of 10 would apply to the worst stuttering the child has produced. The clinician also assigns an SR for the same sample of speech. If there is a discrepancy between the SR of the parent and that of the clinician of more than 1 scale point, the reasons for this are discussed. Parents may also bring recordings of the child's speech to the clinic for the purposes of establishing how well they agree with the clinician for this measure. The clinician and the parent listen to the recording and assign a score, again discussing any discrepancies. The parent uses the scale only in relation to his or her own child's stuttering; it is not necessary for the parent to have heard any other children stuttering to use the scale.

Between clinic visits the parent records the SR for each day, usually on a prepared sheet, and brings the record to the next clinic visit. The clinician then enters the SR for each day onto the data sheet. In Figure 5.1, the SRs for William for each day are represented by filled circles. For Weeks 1 through 3, the SRs were high, although variable, and William's mother had assigned a rating of 10, the highest on the scale, on three occasions during those weeks. By Weeks 4 and 5, a downward trend in SR was apparent. There was a temporary increase in severity during Week 6, which his mother attributed to a disruption in the family due to the death of a relative. Interestingly, by Week 8 William's %SS score in the clinic was very low but SRs for everyday speaking situations remained quite high. This highlights the need to measure stuttering both inside and outside the clinic (Onslow, Harrison, Jones, & Packman, 2002), as without the SR the clinician could have mistakenly believed that William was no longer stuttering. In fact, it was not until Week 13 that both %SS scores and SRs indicated that stuttering was at a very low level both inside and outside the clinic. William commenced Stage 2 of the program in Week 16.

The SR the parent assigns each day may be for an entire day or for a sample of speech of a least 10 minutes duration during the day. In the latter case, the clinician ensures that the parent selects different situations each day. For example, on Monday the speech sample rated may be when the child is playing with a sibling, on Tuesday it may be when visiting with grandparents, and so on for the remainder of the week.

Assigning SRs for different situations is particularly useful if stuttering is highly variable over the day and the parent reports that an SR for a day does not reflect the extreme variability in stuttering that occurs throughout the day. For example, within 1 day the parent might assign SRs of 2 to some periods of speech and SRs of 8 or 9 to others. Consequently it may be difficult to assess whether the child's stuttering is improving, remaining static, or worsening. In such a scenario, the clinician will want to know how severe the child's stuttering is at its worst.

One response to such a situation is for the parent to collect two SRs each day. At the end of the day the parent records one SR that reflects the best period of speech observed all day and another SR that reflects the most severe stuttering observed all day. When these data are displayed graphically, it is typically much easier to see whether stuttering severity is decreasing. It is particularly important to implement this dual SR procedure if a child with highly variable stuttering severity is approaching the transition from Stage 1 to Stage 2.

Sometimes more than one person assigns SRs. For example, the child may spend part of the week in the care of a grandparent, teacher, or friend. If additional people are assigning SRs, it is important that they are adequately trained in the method and that the level of agreement between all parties is satisfactory. If the child is usually brought to the clinic by the mother, the mother is encouraged to discuss and compare ratings with the child's father, if appropriate, so the father can also contribute to the data collection process.

Sometimes the clinician may doubt that the SR the parent brings to the clinic is a true indication of the child's stuttering severity. For example, sometimes a parent may not record an SR at the end of each day, and then records all seven just prior to coming to the clinic. The clinician needs to address these validity issues with the parent and discuss ways of solving the problem.

Sometimes parents are inconsistent in making SR measures, and may even fail to present any SRs for the previous week. This situation poses a dilemma for the clinician who is now faced with making uninformed decisions about how treatment should proceed. It is emphasized here that valid clinical decisions cannot be made in the absence of beyond-clinic stuttering measures, or with only global statements from the parents about the child's stuttering outside. As can be seen from William's speech measures in Figure 5.1, within-clinic speech samples are not necessarily representative of beyond-clinic speech performance. This situation invariably results in the clinician's making "blind" decisions that may or may not be appropriate.

The clinician, therefore, needs to address the problem constructively and discuss with the parent why outside stuttering measures are not being collected and how the parent and clinician can work together to make those ratings happen. Providing the parent with an SR recording sheet or some other type of chart may help, and placing this on the refrigerator with a magnet, for example, may remind the parent to record the SR each day.

Stutters per Minute of Speaking Time

Clinicians do not always require parents to determine stutters per minute of speaking time (SMST), and this measure is not considered essential, as are the SRs and the %SS measures. However, the SMST is helpful when the clinician is concerned about the reliability of the parent's severity ratings and the accuracy of the parent's identification of stuttering. In the latter case, the parent may fail to identify stutters accurately during treatment, being preoccupied with keeping the child interested in the activity. SMST measures can help to focus the parent on stuttering.

To teach parents to make the SMST measure, the clinician requests that the parent make high-quality audiotape recordings of the child speaking in everyday situations and bring them to the clinic. Together the clinician and parent listen to the recordings and identify instances of stuttering. This is helpful for parents who have trouble identifying stuttering. If the parent fails to identify a stutter, the clinician can replay the previous portion of the tape so that they can hear the stutter again. Any disagreement about stuttering can be discussed. It is important to increase the accuracy of identification, because the parent's ability to validly deliver verbal contingencies for stuttering and stutter-free speech depends on it.

The clinician also shows the parent how to measure accumulated speaking time using a stopwatch. The parent practices identifying stutters and measuring accumulated speaking time concurrently on recordings made at home, and then presents these data to the clinician for checking at the next clinic visit. This process continues until good agreement between parent and clinician is achieved.

The Role of Measurement in the Lidcombe Program

It is important to distinguish between the use of stuttering measures for research purposes and their use in the clinic. There are a number of published reports of outcome research for the Lidcombe Program (Lincoln & Onslow, 1997; Lincoln, Onslow, Lewis, & Wilson, 1996; Onslow, Andrews, & Lincoln, 1994; Onslow, Costa, & Rue, 1990). In these reports, stuttering measures were made independently of the treatment process (Packman & Onslow, 1999). Children were regularly audiotape recorded speaking to a family member and to a person who was not a family member, and also covertly. Recordings were made before and after treatment, and stuttering measures were made blind from these recordings by an independent clinician. All parents involved in the studies made the recordings in the same way so that the data for individual children could be grouped and overall statements about the outcome of the program made.

However, stuttering measures are used quite differently in the clinical setting. To provide a valid appraisal of the child's stuttering, measures are made within the clinic by the clinician, and outside the clinic in the child's everyday environment by the parent. Together these within- and beyond-clinic measures play a number of roles in the day-to-day administration of the Lidcombe Program. The most important of these roles are establishing the extent of the problem, informing clinical decision making, specifying treatment goals, quantifying treatment outcomes, and facilitating communication about stuttering. Unlike the use of stuttering measures in research protocols, when these stuttering measures are used in clinical practice, they need to be used flexibly and reviewed regularly to ensure they are fulfilling all of the roles discussed in the following sections.

Establishing the Extent of the Problem

It is well known that the severity of early stuttering is variable across time and across speaking situations (Bloodstein, 1995; Johnson & Associates, 1959; Onslow, Andrews, et al., 1990). Thus, once it is agreed that the child is stuttering, the clinician gathers speech measures within and beyond the clinic to establish the severity, extent, and variability of stuttering. To this end, parents may be asked to bring to the first clinic visits audiotape or videotape recordings of their children speaking at home.

Measurement-Based Decision Making

The Lidcombe Program is behavioral and, as such, its conduct is based on measurement (for a discussion of the application of the principles of behavior therapy to the treatment of stuttering, see Ingham, 1984). First, when the child and parent attend the clinic for the initial visit, the severity of the child's stuttering will be taken into account when deciding when to implement the program (see Chapter 4). For example, it is known that a child whose stuttering is more severe is likely to take longer to complete Stage 1 of the program (Jones, Onslow, Harrison, & Packman, 2000).

Second, stuttering measures play an important role in the Monitoring Program, which occurs if treatment is not implemented immediately (see Chapter 4). During the Monitoring Program, the clinician gathers stuttering measures at regular intervals to ascertain whether natural recovery is taking place.

Third, once treatment has commenced, stuttering measures provide information about the child's response to treatment, both inside and outside the clinic. An investigation of stuttering measures over the first 4 weeks of the program (Onslow et al., 2002; see Box 5.4) indicated that both severity ratings and %SS measures can be expected to reduce over this period, even in children whose stuttering is severe. Lack of improvement in stuttering severity over a number of weeks at any time during Stage 1 indicates to the clinician that the implementation of the program needs to be adjusted. Lack of improvement may indicate that the measures are not valid, or that the parent is not conducting treatment as directed, or that the child does not find the contingencies powerful enough, and so on. In response, the clinician makes changes to the way the treatment is implemented.

Finally, during Stage 2, there are consequences for any increase in stuttering from the entry-level criteria. The parent may reintroduce structured therapy or the parent and child may return to the clinic more frequently.

In summary, then, stuttering measures guide the clinician and parent in tailoring the timing and methods used in each treatment stage to suit each child.

Box 5.4

Onslow, Harrison, Jones, and Packman (2002) examined the clinic files of 141 preschool children who had participated in the Lidcombe Program at the Stuttering Unit, Bankstown Health Service. The children had all been treated within a 5-year period, and the only exclusion criteria were that (a) they had not completed Stage 1 or (b) they had completed Stage 1 in fewer than five clinic visits. The following data were recorded: (a) number of clinic visits required to complete Stage 1; (b) mean parental severity ratings (SR; obtained from the daily ratings) for each of the first 4 weeks of treatment; and (c) the percentage of syllables stuttered (%SS), as scored by the clinician, during the first five clinic visits.

The median number of clinic visits taken to complete Stage 1 was 12. This is slightly higher than previous findings (see Onslow, Andrews, & Lincoln, 1994), because children who completed Stage 1 in fewer than five clinic visits were excluded from the study. Univariate proportional hazards regression showed that the %SS score at Visit 1 and the SR scores reported at Visit 2 strongly predicted number of clinic visits required to complete Stage 1. In other words, children with more severe stuttering, as measured by both %SS and severity ratings, took longer to complete Stage 1 than children whose stuttering was less severe. SR scores were better than %SS scores at predicting time to complete Stage 1. There was moderate and significant correlation between %SS and severity rating scores over the 4 weeks.

SR scores and %SS scores all decreased steadily over the 4 weeks, with the overall decrease being 30%. This decrease occurred for both the mean scores and the upper quartile scores.

Specifying Treatment Goals

The treatment goals of the Lidcombe Program are operationalized in terms of stuttering measures. Progression from Stage 1 to Stage 2 is contingent on the child's stuttering reaching low severity and meeting rate criteria both within and beyond the clinic (see Chapter 7). Thus, it is known at the start of the program that Stage 2 will not commence until stuttering measures reach those criteria. Furthermore, stuttering must continue to meet those speech performance criteria in order for the child to progress through Stage 2.

Quantifying Treatment Outcomes

The gathering of stuttering measures before the program commences and at the conclusion of the program allows the clinician to quantify the outcome of intervention for each child. Such information is essential for accountability to both parents and others who fund stuttering treatments.

Facilitating Communication About Stuttering

Stuttering measures allow for unambiguous communication between the clinician and the parent about stuttering. Rather vague adjectives such as *mild* are replaced by references to data, and vague parental statements such as "I think his stuttering was a bit better this week" are replaced by statements such as "I rated his stuttering at an average of 4 this week, which is better than last week when it was 7." When a parent mentions an SR score, the clinician immediately knows to what stuttering severity the parent is referring.

Conclusion

The Lidcombe Program is a behavioral program and thus incorporates measurement within its procedures. This chapter has discussed the various forms of stuttering measures routinely used in the Lidcombe Program and the important roles that measurement plays in the conduct of the program. What, how, and when speech measures are collected are tailored for each child and family to ensure that the measures truly reflect the child's stuttering inside and outside the clinic and that the measures adequately inform clinical decision making.

References

Bloodstein, O. (1995). *A handbook on stuttering* (5th ed.). San Diego: Singular Publishing Group.

Ingham, R. J. (1984). *Stuttering and behavior therapy: Current status and experimental foundations*. San Diego: College-Hill Press.

Ingham, R. J., & Cordes, A. K. (1992). Interclinic differences in stuttering-event counts. *Journal of Fluency Disorders, 17*, 171–176.

Johnson, W., & Associates. (1959). *The onset of stuttering*. Minneapolis, MN: University of Minneapolis Press.

Jones, M., Onslow, M., Harrison, E., & Packman, A. (2000). Treating stuttering in young children: Predicting treatment time in the Lidcombe Program. *Journal of Speech, Language, and Hearing Research,* 6, 1440–1450.

Lincoln, M., & Onslow, M. (1997). Long-term outcome of an early intervention for stuttering. *American Journal of Speech–Language Pathology,* 6, 51–58.

Lincoln, M., Onslow, M., Lewis, C., & Wilson, L. (1996). A clinical trial of an operant treatment for school-age children who stutter. *American Journal of Speech–Language Pathology*, 5, 73–85.

Onslow, M., Andrews, C., & Costa, L. (1990). Parental severity scaling of early stuttered speech: Four case studies. *Australian Journal of Human Communication Disorders*, 18, 47–61.

Onslow, M., Andrews, C., & Lincoln, M. (1994). A control/experimental trial of an operant treatment for early stuttering. *Journal of Speech and Hearing Research*, 37, 1244–1259.

Onslow, M., Costa, L., & Rue, S. (1990). Direct early intervention with stuttering: Some preliminary data. *Journal of Speech and Hearing Disorders*, 55, 405–416.

Onslow, M., Harrison, E., Jones, M., & Packman, A. (2002). Beyond-clinic speech measures during the Lidcombe Program of early stuttering intervention. *ACQuiring Knowledge in Speech, Language, and Hearing*, 4, 82–85.

Packman, A., & Onslow, M. (1998). The behavioral data language of stuttering. In A. K. Cordes & R. J. Ingham (Eds.), *Treatment efficacy for stuttering: A search for empirical bases* (pp. 27–50). San Diego: Singular Publishing Group.

Packman, A., & Onslow, M. (1999). Recovery from early stuttering: Clarifying some issues. *American Journal of Speech–Language Pathology*, 8, 94–95.

Wingate, M. E. (2001). SLD is not stuttering. *Journal of Speech, Language, and Hearing Research*, 44, 381–383.

Yairi, E., & Ambrose, N. G. (1999). Early childhood stuttering: I. Persistence and recovery rates. *Journal of Speech, Language, and Hearing Research*, 42, 1097–1112.

Chapter 6

Verbal Response-Contingent Stimulation

Mark Onslow

This chapter deals with the application of parental verbal response-contingent stimulation,[1] the fundamental treatment agent of the Lidcombe Program. The term "parental verbal response-contingent stimulation" means that parents say certain things after their children do certain things: the responses. There are two essential responses in the Lidcombe Program: stutter-free speech and unambiguous stuttering. These responses are considered in some detail, as are two nonessential responses that we like to see, and that we encourage, although the Lidcombe Program can occur without them.

Stutter-Free Speech

Stutter-free speech is the most important response to mention. As we reiterate throughout this text, just like any other speech pathology intervention, the Lidcombe Program must be a positive and enjoyable experience for children. One way to ensure that positive and enjoyable experience is for parents to focus during treatment on their children's stutter-free speech far more than on their stuttering. This is absolutely essential for success with the Lidcombe Program. The working rule of thumb is that parents need to highlight stutter-free speech at least five times more often than stuttering. This is particularly the case in the early stages of treatment when there may be considerable stuttering.

In the Lidcombe Program, the language parents use is critical. Various terms are commonly used to describe stutter-free speech, but there are no hard-and-fast guidelines. The point is for the parent to communicate effectively to the child. Commonly, parents use the terms "smooth" or "no bumps" to refer to stutter-free speech with their children. There is, however, no one correct way.

Unambiguous Stuttering

There is much in the current literature to suggest that there are some issues surrounding the identification of stuttering and moments of stuttering in young children. Fortunately, there is no need to cover that literature in the context of the present text, because any child with a clinical diagnosis of stuttering will display many moments of

[1] In this chapter and other places in this text, this term is shortened to "parental verbal contingencies" or "verbal contingencies."

unambiguous stuttering. It is true that some stuttering will be ambiguous to parents (and clinicians). In other words, it may not be clear whether or not some disfluencies are actually stuttering. These ambiguous speech events are not the responses of the Lidcombe Program. Only stutterings that are obviously such to parents attract verbal contingencies. It is critical to note at this stage that every response of stuttering does not attract a parental contingency. In fact, few occasions of stuttering during everyday speech attract contingencies. Stuttering is the only response in the Lidcombe Program for which clinicians and parents attempt to reduce the response rate to zero. All other responses are thought of as desirable, and attempts are made to increase them.

As is the case with stutter-free speech, the language that parents use to describe stuttering is important. Terms commonly used by parents are "bumps," "bumpy," "bumpy word," "stuck," "stuck word," or even "stutter" if it is preferred. Again, the important thing is to choose the term or set of terms that communicate effectively with the child.

Nonessential Responses

Nonessential responses that clinicians using the Lidcombe Program like to see from children, but are not essential to the treatment, include spontaneous self-correction and self-evaluation of speech performance. In a sense, these responses are a bonus, because the treatment can—and does—work if they do not occur. However, we enjoy seeing children demonstrate them, and all the Lidcombe clinicians believe that the treatment is going along particularly well if this occurs. Probably, this reaction is because these responses show that the children have cognitively mastered what the treatment is about and are trying hard to fix their stuttering. On many occasions parents will observe that spontaneous self-correction of stuttering occurs. In other words, the child will stutter and then, without being asked, go back and repeat the utterance or the word without stuttering. Naturally, we encourage parents to reserve special praise for such self-corrections, for example, "Wonderful, you fixed that bump all by yourself."

Another nonessential but desirable response is for the child to self-evaluate speech performance. Children will often be heard to say things such as "I am not doing any bumps any more," or "No bumps today." Again, we encourage parents to reserve special praise for when such self-evaluation occurs. An interesting variation of this response, that does occur sometimes and that is clinically excellent to see, is when the child seeks evaluation from the parent. As reported by one of the parents in Chapter 16, this is likely to occur during Stage 2 of the treatment when the parent may not be continuing to praise stutter-free speech because the stuttering is gone.

Kinds of Parental Verbal Response-Contingent Stimulation

There are four kinds of verbal contingencies from which parents can select when a response occurs. Choosing the right one for use at the right time is important in the Lidcombe Program. It also is important for the clinician to realize that all parents are different and will apply these verbal contingencies in a different way. Figure 6.1 overviews the responses and the parental verbal contingencies in the Lidcombe Program. In short, contingent on stutter-free speech, the parent may acknowledge the response, praise the response, or request a self-evaluation of the response. Con-

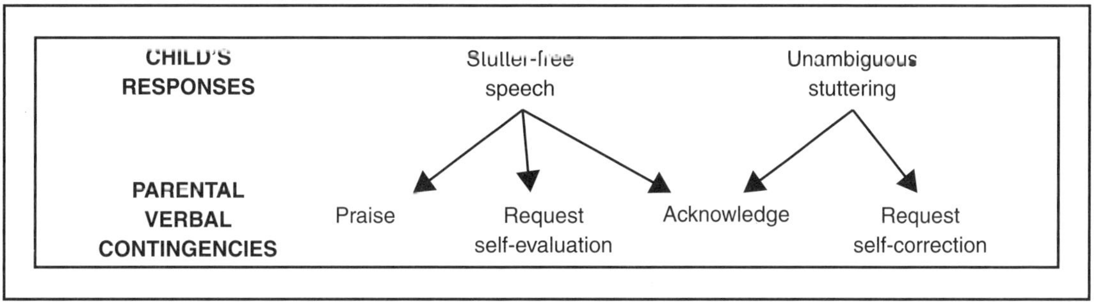

CHILD'S RESPONSES
Stutter-free speech
Unambiguous stuttering
PARENTAL VERBAL CONTINGENCIES
Praise
Request self-evaluation
Acknowledge
Request self-correction

Figure 6.1. The child's responses and the parental verbal contingencies in the Lidcombe Program.

tingent on unambiguous stuttering, the parent may acknowledge the response or request a self-correction of the response In Figure 6.1 and in the text, these verbal contingencies are described individually, but in practice they often occur concurrently. For example, a parent may acknowledge a stutter before requesting self-correction.

Note that parents do not request self-evaluation of stuttered speech in the Lidcombe Program. There are two reasons for this, both of which relate more to clinical common sense than anything else. First, stutter-free speech is the goal of the Lidcombe Program, so it makes sense to align children's self-evaluation with that goal, not with the problem behavior. Second, because self-evaluation is a desirable response in the Lidcombe Program, it makes no sense to associate it with the undesirable response of stuttering.

Acknowledging Stutter-Free Speech and Unambiguous Stuttering

Much of what parents say in the Lidcombe Program is low-key acknowledgment of stutter-free speech and unambiguous stuttering, without any positive evaluation. That is the key to the difference between acknowledgment of the response and praising the response: The former is associated with no words or inflections to suggest that the parent is pleased. All the parent does is quietly and quickly acknowledge that a response has occurred, and the conversation moves on. The following are some examples:

That was smooth.

Smooth talking.

There was a little bump there.

I heard a stuck word.

No bumps.

The advantage of this technique is that it is not disruptive to the flow of conversation. Asking a child to self-correct, as described later, requires that the conversation be stopped momentarily, and praising a child also can be disruptive to the flow of conversation. Of course, such positive input is critical with the Lidcombe Program, as it is with any speech pathology procedure with children. However, praise can be overdone to the point that it becomes meaningless, and even burdensome to the child. Excessive use of praise in the Lidcombe Program often leads to repetitive verbal patterns, which also become meaningless. On many occasions, the parent may simply wish to acknowledge the response in passing. The acknowledgment technique is also useful in the early stages of treatment, when the child is becoming accustomed to what occurs in the Lidcombe Program. Low-key acknowledgment of stutter-free speech and unambiguous stuttering can be a helpful introduction of the procedures to the child.

Praising Stutter-Free Speech

Praising a response is different from acknowledging a response, because it contains positive evaluation of some kind. In praising stutter-free speech, parents typically take a little more time and express real pleasure in what the child has done. It is not a neutral verbal marker, as is acknowledgment of stutter-free speech. The fact that children need the approval of their parents is likely to be one reason that the Lidcombe Program seems to work; children simply enjoy praise from their parents. Praise is applied to stutter-free speech response (and to the responses of spontaneous self-correction and spontaneous self-evaluation if they occur). Examples include the following:

> Lovely smooth talking.
>
> Great! No bumps; that sounded so good.
>
> Lovely, you sounded so smooth then. No bumps at all.
>
> You fixed the bumpy word all by yourself. Good job!

Requesting Self-Evaluation of Stutter-Free Speech

The parent should choose only periods of stutter-free speech for the child to self-evaluate, so the correct evaluation is always that the speech was stutter-free. Examples of requests for self-evaluation include the following:

> Was that smooth?
>
> Were there any bumps there?
>
> Was that bumpy?

Naturally, if the child makes the correct evaluation—that there were no stutters—the parent responds in some clinically appropiate manner, by saying, for example, "Very good," or "Yes, that was smooth."

Requesting Self-Correction of Unambiguous Stuttering

Using the literature on the operant control of stuttering as a guide, we believe that requesting self-correction of stuttering is likely the most powerful treatment agent in the Lidcombe Program (for an overview, see Onslow, 1996). Simply, the parent extends the technique of acknowledging that a stutter has occurred by asking the child to self-correct. A variant of this is to ask whether the child wishes to self-correct. The latter can be an effective approach to determining the child's response to being asked to self-correct. Naturally, if the child declines to self-correct, that response is accepted. There are exceptions to the foregoing rule that parents will know when to apply, but it is a useful rule at the start of the treatment while the parent is becoming accustomed to the procedures. The following are examples:

> That was bumpy. Do you want to try it again?
>
> See if you can say "dog" without the bump.
>
> You had a stuck word. Try it again.

If the child corrects the stutter, the parent responds in some clinically appropriate manner, by saying, for example, "Very good, you got rid of the bumps," or "That's perfect now." Of course, if the child fails to correct the stuttering—as will occur sometimes—the parent still needs to say something encouraging and supportive.

It is important to get the valence and the parental tone right for all the verbal contingencies in the Lidcombe Program, but particularly in the case of requests for self-correction.

There is always the threat that the parent will tend to slip into a negative mode, or convey urgency or anxiety in the way the request for correction is handled. Most parents, with demonstration from the clinician, will intuitively grasp the notion of asking for correction in a positive and supportive manner, but some parents will require careful training. There can also be a tendency for parents to physically gesture to their children that they have stuttered, thereby conveying the opposite of what the clinician intends: that the Lidcombe Program is a helpful, enjoyable, and supportive procedure for the child.

It is essential to let the parent and child find their own way of using all four techniques of contingent verbal stimulation. As noted in Chapter 1, the parent is the expert with the child. If the clinician tries to impose a way of responding verbally in the Lidcombe Program, the parent is likely to feel uncomfortable with the procedure. As has been stressed already, the treatment is individualized for each child, and there are as many ways of doing the Lidcombe Program as there are families with a stuttering preschooler who come to a clinic for help. The treatment relies absolutely on the relation between parents and child, and every such relationship is different, as is every child and every parent. Consequently, every presentation of the Lidcombe Program is different, even though in each case the clinician is attempting to achieve the same thing: parental verbal-contingent stimulation of various responses during everyday conversations.

Treatment in Structured and Unstructured Conversations

Although the clinician is attempting to achieve a situation where the parent acknowledges stuttering and stutter-free speech, praises it, requests self-evaluations of it, and requests corrections of stuttering during everyday conversations, it is not wise to begin the treatment in the conversations of everyday life. For if verbal contingencies are presented thoughtlessly and carelessly by a parent, without adequate training and supervision from the clinician, it can be quite unpleasant for the child. Therefore, the first stage in implementing these verbal contingencies is for the clinician to ensure that parents are presenting verbal contingencies correctly and safely. This occurs by conducting the treatment in structured conversations before conducting it in the unstructured conversations of daily life. This process is described below and overviewed in Figure 6.2.

Treatment in Structured Conversations

During treatment in structured conversations, the Lidcombe clinicians commonly have the parent and child seated at a table or on the floor, engaged in an activity with building blocks, plastic links, a story book, or something similar. When the parent and child are learning about what will happen in the Lidcombe Program, such activities can be useful ways to facilitate association between required responses and verbal contingencies. For example, the parent can couple praise with presentation of a building block or plastic link. The activities can also provide a means to focus and enhance the child's attention, and to generally make the whole procedure fun. During treatment in structured conversations, we often suggest that the parent uses storybooks to elicit conversation from the child.

The clinical commonsense approach in teaching structured conversations to parents is to teach them something positive first. We find that having them acknowledge and praise children's stutter-free speech is a good way to start, and then to introduce acknowledgment of stuttering later in the same clinic visit or

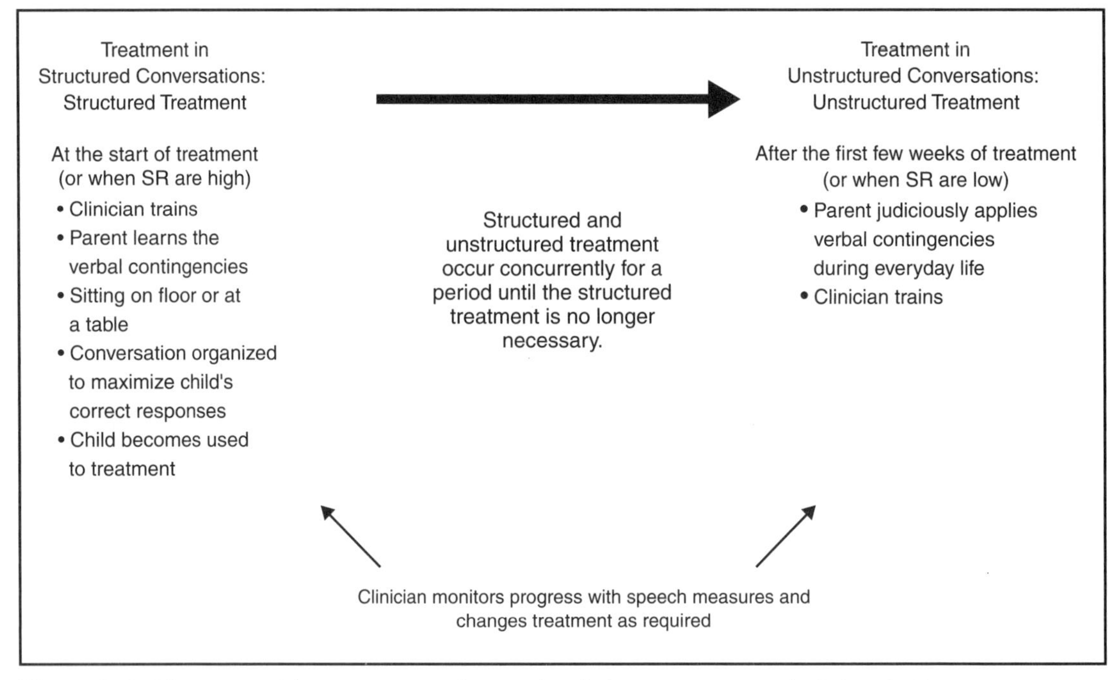

Figure 6.2. The nature of the presentation of parental verbal contingencies in the Lidcombe Program.

during the next clinic visit. Then, last in the learning sequence, the clinician teaches parents how to ask children to self-correct stutters during these structured activities. At this point the clinician and parent need to work closely together to ensure that children enjoy the procedure, and to look out for any signs that children are responding negatively to treatment. Being sure that treatment is presented properly for children is a clinical skill, and it can be a challenge for the clinician to show parents how to do the procedure with children the clinician has known for only a short time (on most occasions parent training for structured conversations begins during the first clinic visit). We find that if the clinician has to "feel around" somewhat to find the right way to present verbal-contingent stimulation to the child, the parent feels more relaxed about attempting the procedure.

The object of structured conversations is to maintain response rate at an optimal level for the child to learn. A rule of thumb, then, is that the child's stuttering rate should stay quite low when parents are giving response-contingent verbal stimulation in structured conversations. By far the most important thing for the clinician to teach parents is to set the task at the correct level of difficulty for the child so that optimal learning occurs. In some situations, the parent will need to elicit single-syllable words from a child, and praise the stutter-free ones, occasionally acknowledging a stutter and asking for self-correction of stuttering. On other occasions, when the child is not stuttering as severely, the parent will elicit a phrase or an utterance or even a considerable period of speech before offering praise. In both situations, the number of stuttered responses should be about the same, so that the overall rate of stuttering is quite low. The most critical thing about giving response-contingent verbal stimulation in structured conversations is for parents to change the difficulty of the task during the conversation as the child improves over the course of it, which virtually always happens. For example, a structured conversation might begin with the parent praising short, stutter-free phrases, and during a matter of minutes, gradually presenting that praise for longer and longer speech segments. Also, during the course of a structured conversation, a parent needs to learn to do the reverse if needed, reverting to praise for shorter utterances.

We normally recommend that sessions occur for 10 to 15 minutes once or twice per day. At some stage during the first weeks of the Lidcombe Program, which are dominated by verbal contingencies in structured conversation, the parent begins to offer praise, acknowledge responses, and request corrections in unstructured situations during everyday life.

Treatment in Unstructured Conversations

Before the introduction of treatment in unstructured conversations, the child will have become comfortable with the kinds of parental verbal contingencies in the Lidcombe Program, will know what is required when a parent asks for a self-correction, and will be generally positive about the treatment. That is the time to introduce the treatment in unstructured conversations. In short, the verbal contingencies that were presented in the structured conversations now switch to occurring during everyday life, and all the structured components are dropped. There is no sitting down at a table with structured activities, and no modifying the conversation so that the child has a high success rate. Simply, during everyday life, in naturally occurring and spontaneous conversations, the parent now begins to praise, to acknowledge responses, and to ask the child to self-correct stuttering. For a period during the Lidcombe Program, treatment in structured conversations and in unstructured conversations occurs concurrently.

In our experience it normally works best for one parent to do the treatment in structured conversations, but for both parents to do the treatment in unstructured conversations. It can be helpful also, with some families, to recruit significant other people who spend time with the child and who are thought to be appropriate, such as grandparents or older siblings, for treatment in unstructured conversations. As was the case with the structured conversations, treatment in unstructured conversations is introduced strategically. This is probably more important than the phasing-in of the full range of parent verbal contingencies during structured conversations, because the treatment moves into everyday life. Obviously, then, it is wise to begin with acknowledgment and praise for stutter-free speech in everyday speaking situations, perhaps followed by acknowledgment of stuttering, and finally requests for self-correction of stuttering.

The moving of the verbal contingencies of the Lidcombe Program from structured conversations into the activities of daily life is a turning point for parents, and can be associated with some apprehension. Praising and acknowledging stutter-free speech and asking for self-correction during the rough-and-tumble of everyday life is much different than doing so during quiet, structured conversations at home. Most noticeably, during structured conversations, many contingencies are presented, and the child and parent are focused exclusively on speech. The situation changes during the introduction of treatment into everyday unstructured conversations. In fact, in one sense, it is essential that this part of treatment is completely dissimilar to the treatment in structured conversations. In everyday life, the parental verbal contingencies are few and far between compared with how often they are presented during structured conversations.

Treatment in unstructured conversations is not simply an extension of treatment during structured conversations. If it is, the treatment will become constant, intensive, and invasive. When such a situation occurs, clinical problems always follow (see Part III). At no point must the child feel that life is permeated with parental responses to speech or that the experience is intense. As noted previously, one common problem is when parents imply something negative in their verbal or nonverbal behavior when requesting self-correction of stuttering during structured conversations. If parents do so continuously during everyday childhood life, clinical disaster quickly follows. Finally, the treatment must not be invasive in the sense that the child's daily communication with family is curtailed, or that the child's relationship with the parent changes in any way.

In both structured and unstructured situations, it is essential for parental verbal contingencies to be presented often. However, in unstructured situations, the parent chooses judiciously when and how often to present contingent verbal stimulation. This process is carefully supervised and regulated by the clinician. Just as parents require training in presenting contingencies in structured conversations, they require training in doing so in unstructured conversation: The clinician demonstrates a technique, then asks the parent to use it, then gives feedback. This process is logistically more taxing than when the child, parent, and clinician are seated at a table or on the floor. One option that should not be excluded is for the three to walk outside the clinic room—even outside in the open air—as the clinician teaches the parent when, how, and how often to acknowledge the child's responses, praise stutter-free speech, and ask for self-correction of stuttering. Under such teaching circumstances, the clinician can see much about how the parent presents the contingencies, which may not be observable in the clinic. For example, the parent may be reluctant to present a contingency for fear of interrupting the child's flow of communication, and the clinician, in a more realistic setting than the clinic, can assist in addressing that issue. In cases where moving outside the clinic is not possible, we often find it helpful for the parent to bring a tape recording of verbal contingencies being presented during unstructured conversations.

The kinds of life situations in which treatment occurs, and how often the parent applies verbal contingencies, must be carefully tailored by the clinician. Because every family is different in terms of personalities, number, schedules, and so on, the way that the treatment is done differs for each. The number of issues that the clinician needs to address in making the treatment occur correctly are numerous, and are dealt with in detail in Chapter 8.

There are only two invariant rules during these early weeks of the treatment in unstructured conversations. First, praise and acknowledgment of stutter-free speech must occur at least five times more than requests for self-correction. Second, the clinical speech measures (see Chapter 5) must show some sign of improvement during the first 5 weeks of treatment. If improvement does not occur, something is most likely going wrong (see Chapter 8) that needs attention from the clinician. That is one of the reasons why clinical speech measures are so important: When the treatment begins, it needs to be effective, and if it is not, the reason for that ineffectiveness needs to be quickly uncovered.

During the first weeks of the Lidcombe Program, treatment occurs in both unstructured and structured conversations. When treatment in structured conversations is no longer needed, it is deleted from the Lidcombe Program, and the treatment thereafter consists solely of parents providing the treatment in the unstructured conversations of daily life. The decision to conclude structured treatment is made when the clinician is sure that (a) the parent is presenting verbal contingencies safely and correctly, (b) the procedure is a positive experience for the child, (c) the child has become familiar with the basic procedures of the Lidcombe Program, and (d) the child has achieved some success. When these four goals have been achieved, then the treatment in structured conversations can cease.

Parents often tell us that their children enjoy the structured conversations and ask to continue them when they are no longer necessary. Parents also ask us whether the structured treatment can be reintroduced into the treatment, if thought necessary, once it has been removed. The answer to both these questions is yes.

Reference

Onslow, M. (1996). *Behavioral management of stuttering*. San Diego: Singular Publishing Group.

Chapter 7

Maintenance of Treatment Effects

Margaret Webber and Mark Onslow

Because relapse is a possibility after treatment for stuttering, the Lidcombe Program incorporates a process designed to ensure that the reductions in stuttering that are apparent at the conclusion of Stage 1 are maintained. Stage 2 is designed to ensure monitoring of the child's speech after Stage 1 so that any signs of relapse can be quickly detected by the parent. In this context, relapse is defined as any increase in stuttering above the speech performance criteria achieved at the conclusion of Stage 1. If relapse is detected, corrective action is taken. Stage 2 is critical to the success of the Lidcombe Program because, as demonstrated later in this chapter, signs of relapse do sometimes appear after Stage 1. We find that one of the worst things that can happen with the Lidcombe Program is that signs of impending relapse go undetected, and a child re-presents to the clinic with stuttered speech some years after it was effectively controlled. That situation is devastating for the child, the parent, and the clinician. Also, the speech performance criteria may take longer to reach again if the re-presentation happens beyond the preschool years, as it often does.

During Stage 1 the parents provide verbal contingencies during everyday conversations. During Stage 2 the parent systematically withdraws those verbal contingencies, under the supervision of the clinician, providing that there are no signs of relapse. Inherent in this process is the empowering of parents by giving them full responsibility for the continued monitoring of stuttering. It is not desirable for clinicians to have parents and children depending on them for the maintenance of stutter-free speech.

The Empirical Basis of Stage 2

The fundamental procedures in Stage 2 draw on Ingham's (1980) demonstration of maintenance of treatment effects as a response in therapy, to which contingencies can be applied.[1] One of the contingencies for maintenance of speech criteria applied by Ingham is increasingly longer periods between clinic visits and assessments. If the maintenance response does not occur, then the client returns to a schedule of more frequent visits.

In adapting Ingham's (1980) procedure to Stage 2 of the Lidcombe Program, there is one important difference. Essentially, in Ingham's procedure, it is reinforcing for clients not to have to come to the clinic so often, because those visits are associated with quite a heavy workload of preparing beyond-clinic tapes and talking for long periods to the clinician. However, children enjoy coming to see

[1] One of the most recent versions of Ingham's (1980) procedure is recorded in Ingham (1999).

the clinician during the Lidcombe Program, so it is not rewarding for them not to come. Nonetheless, parents and their children come to the clinic less and less as successful maintenance occurs, with a schedule of visits at increasingly long intervals as outlined later. The most important factor in Ingham's maintenance procedure—the use of stuttering measures to specify criterion speech performance—is also a feature of the Lidcombe Program. That is the most basic concept in Stage 2: The child progresses through Stage 2 if, and only if, speech performance criteria are met.

When To Start Stage 2

The decision about when to start Stage 2 is based primarily on speech measures within and beyond the clinic. The parent and clinician have been collecting stuttering measures throughout the treatment process (see Chapters 1 and 5), and when the program speech criteria are met, it is time to consider beginning Stage 2. Apart from the criterion speech measures listed below, there are additional considerations. First, the child should meet these criteria for 3 weeks before progressing to Stage 2, so the clinician can be certain that stuttering really is under control. The clinician and parent may choose to wait for a longer period of stability if the child's stuttering has been unusually variable during the treatment period. Second, the clinician must be convinced that the speech measures are indeed valid. At this stage of the treatment, the clinician will be fairly confident that this is the case, because the measures have been used throughout Stage 1 (see Chapters 1 and 5), but this point in treatment is so important that it is worth a last check.

Speech criteria for entry into Stage 2 are as follows:

- Severity ratings (SRs) for each day of the week are 1 or 2, with at least four of these being 1.
- Percentage of syllables stuttered (%SS) within the clinic is below 1.0.
- Stutters per minute of speaking time (SMST), if it has been incorporated into the treatment (see Chapter 5), is below 1.5.

The clinician may also decide to ensure that %SS is below 1.0 on a beyond-clinic tape recording made during the previous week. During the last clinic visits of Stage 1, when the clinician and parent need to be absolutely sure that the child's speech warrants the start of Stage 2, it is useful for them both to listen to a 5- to 10-minute beyond-clinic recording of the child while monitoring together for any stutters. On some occasions, particularly with children who do not meet program criteria on a few occasions during Stage 2, we add the below 1%SS criterion to beyond-clinic tape recordings as well as for the child's speech in the clinic. On many occasions, however, during Stage 2 the clinician is confident that the parental SRs and anecdotal reports accurately reflect the child's speech status, and decides that beyond-clinic tape recordings are not needed.

Implementing Stage 2

In practice, the clinician starts to prepare the parent for the implementation of Stage 2 at the start of treatment. When the treatment is being outlined initially to the parent, the clinician explains what will occur when stuttering reaches the low program criteria. As the child nears the end of Stage 1, this discussion with the parent is revisited. We find that this preparation is essential to avoid having parents believe that Stage 2 is merely an add-on rather than an integral part of treatment. As stated earlier, it is extremely problematic when Stage 2 is not implemented correctly and the child relapses. In the worst case scenario, the parent simply stops attending the clinic at the completion of Stage 1. To give the child and the parents the best chance of achieving long-term control of stuttering, the clinician alerts the parent to the importance of Stage 2 of the program throughout Stage 1.[2]

As indicated previously, a schedule of visits is prescribed, with increasing periods between them. In our experiences (see our file audit in the next section of text), around half of the problems that occur during Stage 2 occur during the first 9 weeks. This is one reason why we think it is essential for the first visits during Stage 2 to occur quite close together. The visits are organized with the first two visits 2 weeks apart, then two visits 4 weeks apart, then another two visits 8 weeks apart, and the final visit 16 weeks later. A child progresses through this sequence of visits if criterion speech performance is maintained. Whether or not this has been achieved is determined in a manner similar to the measurement procedures in Stage 1, namely from a %SS measure gathered by the clinician and from the daily parental SRs made during the previous week. If the program criterion speech performance is not achieved at any visit during Stage 2, the clinician decides either to stall progress through the sequence or to return the family to an earlier stage of the sequence. Although the sequencing of visits is not flexible in Stage 2, the action taken in the event of failure to attain criterion speech performance is. It may be considered appropriate for some children to return to the first visit in Stage 2, whereas the clinician may not think this is necessary for other children. This clinically flexible approach to Stage 2 includes ad hoc visits to the clinic between the scheduled visits if necessary (as described later).

As discussed in the next section, in many cases a child will not meet program criteria at one visit during Stage 2. In most of these cases, only one repeat visit will be necessary. However, in a small number of cases, children will require a return to Stage 1, particularly if other strategies to maintain treatment gains are not successful. Life events (e.g., family holidays, a new baby in the family, or illness) can affect progress through Stage 2.

It is important that the clinician manages the parent's systematic withdrawal of verbal contingencies during Stage 2. With stuttering at very low levels or nonexistent at the end of Stage 2, there will be few parental verbal contingencies for stuttering, and the majority of what parents do will be acknowledging and praising stutter-free speech. Often, the clinician's first task at the start of Stage 2 is to ensure that the parent simply does not forget about doing the treatment.

The clinician generally arranges for the parental verbal contingencies to be withdrawn systematically and gradually, providing that no signs of stuttering reappear. When the stuttering is under control, it makes no sense to remove the treatment agent abruptly. As with most other things about the Lidcombe Program, the way this is done is individualized for each family. In general, though, two principles are used. The first is that the clinician relies on information provided at each clinic visit in making decisions about the rate at which verbal contingencies are withdrawn—that is, whether to slow the process down, speed it up, or keep it going at the same rate. The second principle is that by the end of Stage 2 the stuttering should be at a very low level or nonexistent, without any verbal contingencies at all, but with the parent ready to introduce them if needed. There is some flexibility here, however, and in some cases the clinician may think it desirable for the contingencies to continue after the completion of Stage 2. Withdrawal of contingencies can be managed systematically. For example, a clinician may instruct the parent, during 1 month, to present the verbal contingencies on 6 days per week, with none on the remaining day. During the next month the parent presents the verbal contingencies on 5 days per week, and so on.

[2] As indicated in Chapter 1, we prefer the term "Stage 2" to "maintenance" because it conveys that this is part of the treatment and not an add-on.

When Stage 2 begins, parents are skilled at presenting verbal contingencies in structured and unstructured conversations, and the clinician advises them that, if any signs of stuttering appear, they should respond as appropriate with those skills. The clinician advises the parent that prompt action is important, and not to wait for the next Stage 2 visit, which could be up to 6 months away. The usual appropriate response of a parent in the event of signs of an increase in stuttering would be to increase or reintroduce verbal contingencies in unstructured conversations. If needed, the parent can reintroduce the contingencies in structured conversations as well. This is a conservative approach to the problem, but it will not do any harm.

Parents need to evaluate the effect of any action they take and make adjustments accordingly, as they did during Stage 1. We find it is important here, as in any part of the Lidcombe Program, for parents to be aware how easy it is to slip into just asking the children for self-correction of stuttering and to forget to provide contingencies for stutter-free speech. At this point it may be necessary to remind the parent of the rule of thumb in the Lidcombe Program that if they have asked a child to self-correct stuttering, then they need to use contingencies for stutter-free speech a number of times before correcting again. During Stage 1 the rule of thumb is a ratio of at least five instances of reinforcement of stutter-free speech for each correction of stuttering. However, clinicians can be less prescriptive during Stage 2, because the parents at this stage are completely aware of the issues with presenting verbal contingencies to their children, and are unlikely to overdo the correction.

In implementing Stage 2, the parent needs to know what access to the clinician can be expected outside the scheduled visits. One purpose of Stage 2 is to empower parents to manage their child's stuttering themselves, but we are aware of the need not to require too much too soon. Consequently, the clinician may suggest that the parent phone at any time during business hours to discuss any problems that arise. If necessary, clinic visits can be arranged between scheduled Stage 2 visits, but the need for this does not arise often.

A Clinical File Audit of Stage 2

At the Stuttering Unit, Bankstown Health Service, Sydney, files of 25 children were accessed. These were cases that were admitted to Stage 2 after achieving criterion speech performance in the usual manner. The sample contained 17 boys and 8 girls. Mean age at entry to Stage 1 was 42 months (range: 2 years 7 months to 4 years 10 months) and mean age at entry to Stage 2 was 52 months (range: 3 years 4 months to 5 years 9 months). The mean %SS measure at the first Stage 1 visit was 4.4 (range: 1.2 to 19.0%SS). The clinical files were audited to determine the number of occasions on which the children did not meet program criteria on at least one scheduled Stage 2 visit.

Ten of the children did not achieve criterion speech performance at one Stage 2 visit, and 3 of the children did not achieve criterion speech performance at two visits. This means that 13 (52%) of the children showed some evidence of reappearance of their stuttering after Stage 1, and there was a total of 16 occasions of failure to meet program criteria at a Stage 2 visit. In 4 of these cases (3 boys and 1 girl), the clinician decided to return the child and parent to Stage 1 and to reenter Stage 2 when performance criteria had been met for a second time. During this second attempt at Stage 2, 3 of the 4 children met program criteria at each visit, and 1 progressed through Stage 2 only failing to meet program criteria at one visit. For the 16 occasions when children did not meet program criteria at a visit during Stage 2, the mean period that this occurred was 7 weeks after the start of Stage 1 (range: 1 to 24 weeks). Twelve of the 16 occasions occurred within 8 weeks after the start of Stage 2.

For all cases in which program criteria were not met, other than those that resulted in a return to Stage 1, the parent reintroduced or increased the rate of verbal contingencies in unstructured conversations. In 4 of the 16 occasions in which criterion perfomance was not met, the clinician instructed the parent to reintroduce verbal contingencies in structured conversations as well. On most occasions, repeated visits were scheduled for 1 or 2 weeks later. In the case of 3 children, the clinician's file notes indicated that parents successfully managed the signs of increasing stuttering without needing to contact the clinic, merely reporting the incident during the scheduled Stage 2 visit.

In 24 (96%) of the files surveyed, the clinicians made notes about the parents' use of verbal contingencies during Stage 2. In all these cases, it was noted that children began Stage 2 with parents continuing to present verbal contingencies in unstructured conversations. In 5 (21%) of these 24 cases, the parents were still doing some treatment in structured conversation at the start of Stage 2; however, these were all phased out during the first few weeks of Stage 2. Clinicians' notes showed that, in all cases, the rate at which verbal contingencies in unstructured conversations were withdrawn varied considerably. In most cases, no contingencies were used at the second last visit; however, 4 children were reported to be receiving some limited verbal contingencies in unstructured conversations at the completion of Stage 2.

In summary, these are the clinically important findings about Stage 2 to emerge from this file audit:

- In all cases, parents were presenting verbal contingencies at the start of Stage 2.
- In around 20% of cases, parents were presenting verbal contingencies in structured conversations at the start of Stage 2, but these practices stopped within a few weeks.
- In most cases, verbal contingencies were not being used by parents at the conclusion of Stage 2.
- Stage 2 requires around 12 months on average to complete.
- In around 50% of children, there will be a visit during Stage 2 at which the child does not meet program criteria, at which time clinical action is required.
- Most of these occasions can be managed effectively, and it is rare for children to need to be returned to Stage 1.
- Seventy-five percent of the occasions on which program criteria were not met occurred within 8 weeks of the start of Stage 2.
- A common and effective management strategy when children do not meet program criteria during Stage 2 is for parents to reintroduce or increase the rate of verbal contingencies in unstructured conversation.

A Typical Stage 2 Clinic Visit

As indicated previously, the primary purpose of the Stage 2 clinic visit is to assess the child's speech with reference to program criteria, and to determine whether the child progresses to the next scheduled visit. In making this decision, the clinician relies on Lidcombe Program speech measures but also draws on sources of information beyond those measures. The clinician needs to be continually alert for the appearance of any sources of unreliability or threats to the validity of those speech measures. The success of the entire treatment may depend on such problems being detected and fixed. For example, the parent may lose interest during Stage 2 and become careless and nonvigilant when making SRs, believing mistakenly (as stated earlier) that there is no risk that stuttering will reappear.

As with clinic visits during Stage 1, the visit starts with the clinician collecting a within-clinic measure of %SS. The clinician then records the parental SRs made for each day of the week prior to the visit, and the SMST scores if they have been collected (see Chapter 5). If presented, the beyond-clinic recording is also rated for %SS. Again, using standard procedures for a Lidcombe Program visit, we use these measures as a focus of a discussion about what has happened since the last visit. This allows parents the opportunity to bring up any relevant issues or problems. As stated at the start of this chapter, one of the purposes of Stage 2 is to empower parents by finally transferring to them the responsibility of managing their child's stuttering. Therefore, the aim of this initial discussion at each Stage 2 clinic visit is to encourage parents (a) to analyze any problems that have emerged since the last visit, (b) to establish fresh insights into the problems, and (c) to formulate their own solutions to them.

Because SRs are so important in Stage 2, the clinician pays particular attention to how the parent is collecting them. In particular, the clinician is vigilant for any changes in the judgments parents are making that underpin their scores. For example, parents may change from basing their ratings on an entire day to basing them on a particular period during the day. If that occurs, it is important for the clinician to know it. Furthermore, Stage 2 is a time when "drift" may occur in the way that the parent assigns severity ratings to the child's speech. For example, the parent may begin to react inappropriately to normal disfluencies. As always in the Lidcombe Program, it is important to "calibrate" the parent's SR against a within-clinic %SS score. The procedure for doing this is simply to ask the parent to assign an SR to the speech on which the clinician's %SS score is based (see Chapter 5). Any problems with the appropriateness of the parental severity score can easily be detected with this method.

The parent and clinician decide if the child's speech measures meet the program criteria, and they decide when the next visit will occur, either the next in the prescribed Stage 2 sequence or some other scheduled visit according to need. As the results of the file audit described earlier show, in cases where criterion speech performance is not met, the most common clinical response is to reschedule the visit 1 or 2 weeks later. As with all clinic visits in the Lidcombe Program, the session ends with the clinician outlining what the parent should be aiming to achieve in the period until the next visit. When criterion speech performance has been achieved, that outline will focus on whether verbal contingencies should be systematically withdrawn and, if so, how they should be withdrawn. In the event of criterion speech performance not being met, these directions most commonly focus on increasing the rate of verbal contingencies in unstructured conversations, or reintroducing verbal contingencies in structured conversations, or perhaps a combination of both.

Two Case Studies of Stage 2

Martin: A Routine Case

Martin was age 3 years 4 months when he began Stage 1 of the Lidcombe Program, and required 11 weeks to reach Stage 2. His schedule of Stage 2 visits and speech criteria were standard as outlined previously in this chapter. At the time he entered Stage 2, his mother was acknowledging and praising stutter-free speech in unstructured conversations. The clinician advised his mother to take 3 to 4 months to gradually withdraw these verbal contingencies if Martin continued to meet the program stuttering criteria.

At Martin's first Stage 2 visit, all speech measures—SRs and %SS—showed no stuttering. Martin's mother reported giving intermittent praise for stutter-free speech during the previous fortnight. The clinician advised Martin's mother to continue to gradually withdraw this over the coming months. Martin and his mother were unable to attend the next visit in 2 weeks, so this second clinic visit was arranged for 3 weeks later.

At the second Stage 2 visit, Martin's mother reported that all severity ratings were 1 during the previous week. However, she observed occasional stuttering on 2 days since the last visit. In response to this, she reported that she increased the frequency of praise for stutter-free speech and asked Martin to correct the stutters; she observed no further stuttering. The clinician observed no stuttering in the clinic and praised the mother's early detection of, and subsequent response to, the stuttering. The clinician arranged the next visit for 4 weeks later. The clinician recommended that the mother continue to give praise at the current rate for another 2 weeks before reducing it again.

At the third Stage 2 visit, Martin's mother reported no stuttering during the previous 4 weeks and reported that she no longer provided any verbal contingencies. The clinician observed no stuttering within the clinic. The mother reported that the family would be on vacation at the date of the next scheduled visit, so the clinician and mother decided to schedule the next visit in 8 weeks.

The fourth visit was canceled due to illness in Martin's family, and phone contact was made during the next week in place of clinic visit. The mother reported all SRs were 1. The next visit was arranged for 8 weeks later.

Martin attended for two more visits, and at each of these his mother again reported that SRs were all 1 and the clinician observed no stuttering on requested beyond-clinic tapes and within the clinic. Martin was discharged and the clinician encouraged the mother to contact the clinic should she have any concerns about his speech.

John: A Case Illustrating Return to Stage 1 and Reentry to Stage 2

John was age 4 years 5 months when he commenced Stage 1. He had previously attended another clinic for treatment, which had been unsuccessful. John required 20 sessions to complete Stage 1. At the time of entering Stage 2, John's mother gave intermittent acknowledgment and praise for stutter-free speech and praise for spontaneous self-correction of stuttered speech in everyday conversation. Spontaneous self-correction of stuttered speech occurred on the few occasions on which stuttering occurred.

John's speech criteria were the routine ones mentioned previously, and visits were scheduled in the routine weekly intervals: 2, 2, 4, 4, 8, 8, and 16. The clinician recommended that, during the first 2 weeks of Stage 2, John's mother provide treatment exactly as during the last week of Stage 1.

John was unable to attend the clinic for his first Stage 2 visit. His mother made phone contact and reported that his SRs had increased to 4s and 5s in the last half of the week. She reported reintroducing treatment in structured conversations, but reported that this had no effect on John's speech during everyday conversation. The clinician suggested two treatments in structured conversations per day. A visit was arranged for the following week.

John attended this visit and was stutter-free in the clinic. John's mother reported that John's SRs were down to 2 and 3 and that his speech in the clinic at that time was representative of his speech all morning. She reported that John was aware of his recent increase in stuttering and seemed reluctant to do treatment in structured conversations and comply with requests for self-correction. The clinician made the following recommendations:

- Increase the amount of acknowledgment and praise for stutter-free speech
- Use minimal requests for self-correction of stuttering
- Use the contingencies for stutter-free speech system more consistently
- Use treatment in structured conversations only during periods when some SRs increase to 3

At the next clinic visit, the clinician noted that John's mean SR had decreased, although it was still greater than 2.0. Therefore, a repeat visit was scheduled for 2 weeks later. John and his mother were unable to attend his third visit. John's mother reported by telephone that SRs during the previous 2 weeks were all 1s and 2s. She reported following the clinician's recommendations, using much acknowledgment and praise for stutter-free speech in unstructured conversations, and doing some treatment in structured conversations. She also provided occasional tangible reinforcers. The clinician recommended that John's mother maintain all those activities to the same extent until a visit in 2 weeks that was scheduled over the telephone. The clinician asked John's mother to bring a 5-minute tape recording of John's conversational speech to the next clinic visit.

John attended the clinic for his fourth visit and again he was stutter-free in the clinic and on the beyond-clinic tape. John's mother reported SRs of 2 and 1. However, she reported an occasional sound prolongation during the previous week, and the clinician noted that an SR of 2 would not normally occur if the child was prolonging sounds (1 = *very mild stuttering*). The clinician advised John's mother to continue with the treatment as previously recommended and to watch closely for any prolongations. John's mother was advised to ask John to self-correct the prolongations but also to maintain an emphasis on acknowledgment and praise for stutter-free speech. A further visit was arranged for the following week.

At this visit John's mother reported SRs of 2 and 1 except for 1 day where she assigned a 3, essentially because of a period after kindergarten when she observed a number of sound prolongations. The clinician did not observe any of these during the clinic visit; however, a number of part-word repetitions were noted. The clinician decided to return John to Stage 1, and he and his mother subsequently attended weekly treatment for 5 weeks before reentering Stage 2.

At the time of reentering Stage 2, John's SRs were all at the program criterion of 1 and 2. John's mother was providing verbal contingencies intermittently whenever she was with him, and used a tangible reward usually twice each week. The schedule of visits was again set at weekly intervals of 2, 2, 4, 4, 8, 8, and 16. The clinician advised John's mother to reduce the use of the tangible rewards over the next month before starting to reduce verbal contingencies.

At John's first two visits, his mother reported that she continued to give intermittent verbal contingencies as needed and had stopped using tangible rewards. The clinician observed no stuttering in the clinic or on the beyond-clinic tape that John's mother brought to the clinic. John met all Stage 2 speech criteria and the third visit was scheduled 4 weeks later. At the third visit, John's mother reported that she was not hearing any stuttering at home and John's SRs were all 1. She reported still giving occasional acknowledgment and praise for stutter-free speech. The clinician observed no stuttering in the clinic or on the beyond-clinic tape. The next visit was scheduled for 4 weeks later.

John was unable to attend the fourth visit and phone contact was substituted. John's mother mailed the beyond-clinic tape to the clinician. She reported that SRs for the previous week were all 1 and that she praised stutter-free speech once during that week. The clinician advised John's mother to continue to reduce the praise gradually. The next scheduled visit was for 8 weeks later, providing that the mailed beyond-clinic tape met the program criterion of below 1%SS. When the tape was received, the clinician observed no stuttering on it and returned it to John's mother with confirmation of the date of the next visit.

John and his mother attended the clinic for his fifth visit, and his mother reported assigning an SR of 1 for each day of the previous week, and that she no longer provided any verbal contingencies. John's speech was stutter-free in the clinic. John's mother did not bring a beyond-clinic tape as requested by the clinician. John and his mother attended the final two visits, during which John's speech met all program criteria and his mother reported no further problems of any kind. John had completed Stage 2 and was discharged. The clinician encouraged John's mother to contact the clinic should she have any further concerns about his speech.

Transcript of a Videorecording of a Clinician Explaining Stage 2 to a Parent

PARENT: Once you can safely say you've got rid of it (stuttering), what are the chances of it reoccurring?

CLINICIAN: That's a good question. The point where you finish the first part of therapy—Stage 1—is when his severity ratings are mostly 1s and the occasional 2, over a few weeks. So things have been pretty stable, say over 3 weeks, with lots of 1s and an odd 2.

PARENT: Mmm.

CLINICIAN: That's when we consider that he doesn't really need weekly clinic visits anymore. But you're right; by then, even though he doesn't need to see me every week, if you stop doing all the treatment that you're doing at home, it's possible his stuttering would start to increase again. And in fact that's what does happen sometimes. So when his weekly clinic visits finish, we don't say that's the end and stop doing all that you're doing. What will happen is that you will go into Stage 2.

PARENT: Mmm.

CLINICIAN: What Stage 2 is designed to do is to make sure that he continues to talk like that for months and months into the future. And Stage 2 goes on for about a year usually.

PARENT: Oh, right.

CLINICIAN: What it basically involves is clinic visits that are gradually reduced in their frequency. So he'd come in after a fortnight and a fortnight again and then after a month and then a month again. And gradually they get further apart and the last visits might be 4 months apart.

PARENT: Right.

CLINICIAN: And in that time you continue to do what you're doing already at home. So if he gets to the end of Stage 1 and his severity ratings are mostly 1s and you're giving him treatment in everyday conversation at home and it's mostly praising stutter-free speech, and say we start Stage 2 today. Then you would continue to do all those same things at home.

PARENT: Right.

CLINICIAN: Over the next weeks and months, you'll just gradually stop doing them as often, simply because his speech is so good. It's like a natural withdrawal of the treatment.

PARENT: Yes.

CLINICIAN: So by the end of Stage 2, about 12 months down the track, you'll find you probably won't need to be giving any more treatment or you might occasionally praise him for sounding so good.

PARENT: Right.

CLINICIAN: Basically what's happened is you have been trained to become his therapist. The focus of therapy is on what happens at home so even when he finishes coming to Stage 2 visits you'll still know what to do. And if at any time after that you become, for any reason, concerned about his speech, just ring and say what's happening and we'll see you straight away.

PARENT: I see.

CLINICIAN: Just going by the comments of other parents with children just like Michael who go through treatment in a fairly straightforward sort of way and then go to Stage 2, it often happens that—it might be say 2 months into Stage 2—they do have some stuttering, a little relapse. But the relapses are little because straight away you know what to do. So even if it's between visits—it might be he's not coming in for another month—and you notice a few stutters again, you know immediately what to do. You don't have to wait to come back. You just start giving him the appropriate treatment straight away.

PARENT: So you deal with it straight away.

CLINICIAN: And when you come back a few weeks later down the track, you say he did have a relapse and this is what I did about it and this is how it worked. This is often how it goes if there is a relapse.

References

Ingham, R. J. (1980). Modification of maintenance and generalization during stuttering treatment. *Journal of Speech and Hearing Research*, *23*, 723–745.

Ingham, R. J. (1999). Performance-contingent management of stuttering in adolescents and adults. In R. F. Curlee (Ed.), *Stuttering and related disorders of fluency* (2nd ed., pp. 200–221). New York: Thieme Medical.

Chapter 8

Troubleshooting

Elisabeth Harrison, Kerry Ttofari, Isabelle Rousseau, and Cheryl Andrews

Some clinical guides and instruction manuals may be written in a cookbook format; ingredients and quantities are listed, along with directions for combining them. Each treatment application is identical, and success depends on the program being used according to instruction. The cookbook format, however, is not right for the Lidcombe Program. We could include ingredients—the component parts—to be used with all clients, but quantities of those components and the method of combining them differ from client to client. The Lidcombe Program is applied in a unique manner that is optimal for each child and parent. This means that there are as many variations of applications of the Lidcombe Program as there are parents and children who use the treatment.

In addition to reading this text, program users can access information from various sources. The clinical manual may be downloaded from the Web site of the Australian Stuttering Research Centre (http://www.fhs.usyd.edu.au/ASRC/). Lidcombe Program workshops are available regularly in Australia, the United Kingdom, and Canada, taught by local clinicians in each case. In Australia, speech pathologists can also access the Stuttering Unit's consultation service for advice about using the program. Several forms of consultation are used—consultations by telephone, clinic visits to the Stuttering Unit, and e-mail. The Stuttering Unit's consultation service helps clinicians to solve problems that arise while using the Lidcombe Program. Those consultations therefore are a useful source of information about problems that can occur while using the treatment. A study was designed to document the content of Stuttering Unit phone consultations and to establish the most common problems that occur while using the treatment.

Method

Participants

Over a 15-month period, Stuttering Unit clinicians conducted 60 telephone consultations concerning preschool-age children's stuttering treatment using the Lidcombe Program. To avoid confusion, we will refer to those who requested the consultations as *clinicians* and the Stuttering Unit clinicians as *consulting clinicians*.

Consulting clinicians kept notes during each consultation that included each client's age and gender, a brief description of the presenting problem, and advice given to the clinician. These notes were kept to provide a reference to be used if subsequent consultations were requested regarding the client.

Procedure

The second author (Kerry Ttfofari) interviewed the clinicians. Each interview was audiotaped and transcribed. Consulting clinicians referred to their clinical notes when describing each consultation. The names of clinicians were not disclosed to the interviewer. The consulting clinicians reported presenting problems as originally described by the clinician, the contributing problems identified during the course of the consultation, and recommendations given on each occasion.

Analysis

The second author scanned each transcript and coded all information. This preliminary examination indicated that the information could usefully be analyzed in two ways. First, clinicians reported primary reasons that prompted each consultation. These were the reasons given by clinicians when they telephoned the Stuttering Unit, and they are reported in Analysis 1. Second, the consulting clinicians also reported factors that were identified during the course of each consultation as having contributed to the initial problem. These are reported in Analysis 2.

Results

Analysis 1

Reasons given by the consulting clinicians for the consultations fell into two categories: (1) lack of treatment progress and (2) client issues that influence treatment outcome. Of the 60 consultations, 40 (66%) were prompted by slow progress or lack of progress while using the Lidcombe Program. Lack of progress was described more specifically as the range of the child's severity ratings (SRs) remaining stable over many weeks. In 58% of these cases, the consultation was taking place more than 1 year after treatment started. Some clinicians reported cases in which the child's stuttering had been stable for several months. For the remaining 42% of cases, between four and nine clinic visits had occurred before the consultation was requested. There was no common level of stuttering severity at which clients' progress ceased. Some children's treatment progress stopped at a mild severity level, whereas others stabilized at SRs as high as 7.

Regarding client issues that influence treatment, 20 consultations (33%) were initiated by clinicians seeking advice on unusual client-related issues. Although indirectly related to stuttering, these issues had the potential to complicate treatment progress. For example, cases were presented in which children had other communication problems in addition to stuttering. Their clinicians were unsure how to approach treatment and requested advice on how the presence of additional communication problems may affect treatment outcome.

Other clinicians sought advice on how to use the Lidcombe Program with children whose stuttering was marked by characteristics that were unfamiliar to them, such as extremely severe stuttering, blinking while stuttering, or speaking with an odd-sounding, high-pitched voice. Other consultations included requests for advice about using the program with twins, suggestions on how to begin treatment with a 2-year-old who had been stuttering for a short time, treating a child who stuttered more severely in the clinic than at home, and conducting treatment with children who had had previous unsuccessful treatment with other clinicians.

Analysis 2

The second analysis included each of the 60 consultations used in Analysis 1. All consultations were inspected again from the perspective of consulting clinicians. Specifically, this analysis looked for issues that consulting clinicians identified as *contributing* to the presenting problems listed in Analysis 1. Sixteen problems and issues were identified in Analysis 2, and they fell into three categories: (1) problems directly related to application of the Lidcombe Program, (2) parent- and child-related issues that were considered to be hindering treatment progress, and (3) child-related factors not directly related to the Lidcombe Program.

In the following sections, under the three category headings, are listed each of the 16 problems and issues that consulting clinicians identified as contributing to presenting problems. Following brief descriptions of problems and issues are suggested approaches to dealing with them. These suggestions are examples of advice given by consulting clinicians during their discussions with clinicians.

Category 1: Problems Directly Related to Application of the Lidcombe Program

Speech Measures. Consulting clinicians reported that problems with speech measures were present in 14% of consultations. Some parents did not collect SRs or collected them infrequently. In other consultations it became clear that clinicians may have contributed to the problem by failing to communicate to parents the importance of speech measures, or by failing to use the measures to guide treatment. A second reason for parents' inconsistent or non-collection of SRs was identified as lack of training by clinicians.

Some clinicians raised doubts about the reliability of parents' SRs. One clinician reported that a parent described consistent reduction in the child's stuttering, although there was no reduction in the parent's reported SRs.

Suggestions

- During the first weeks of Stage 1, the clinician and parent compare SRs on samples of the child's speech during clinic visits. This allows the clinician to assess how the parent uses the SR scale, and to what extent the parent accurately identifies the child's stutter-free and stuttered speech.
- If SRs do not decrease over several weeks, that does not necessarily indicate a problem. The clinician can look at how the parent conducts treatment in structured conversations. If the child's stutter-free responses are more frequent or utterance length is increasing, then progress is being made.
- Ask the parent if he or she knows why SRs are not decreasing, despite treatment occurring regularly and correctly. For example, the parent may be aware of decreases in the child's stuttering that are not reflected in SRs. This is most likely to occur when the child stutters either severely or very mildly. Despite the reason for SRs not changing, this is an opportunity for the parent and clinician to consult about treatment and progress.

Training Parents. Whereas the problems discussed previously pertain only to measurement, the Lidcombe Program also requires parents to learn other skills, such as linking speech measures and treatment, and presenting treatment consistently. Problems related to training parents were identified in 14% of consultations.

Despite verbal and written instructions to parents, clinicians reported that parental verbal contingencies were presented too slowly or too quickly, or parents were unsure about how to conduct treatment. In all cases, treatment was delivered incorrectly, and the children progressed very slowly or not at all.

Clinicians reported situations in which several family members delivered treatment at home, although only one attended clinic visits and was trained to use the Lidcombe Program. Similar scenarios involved children treated by a parent and another member of the extended family, and children who lived in two households as a result of their parents' separation.

Suggestions

- During clinic visits, especially early in Stage 1, both parent and clinician need to demonstrate treatment. The purpose of this is to provide a platform for consultation and discussion about the child's responsiveness to treatment. Such discussion and consultation between parent and clinician typically last for at least half of each 1-hour clinic visit.
- The clinician needs to observe verbal contingencies for stutter-free and stuttered speech being used by all relatives and caregivers who take responsibility for treatment with the child. Although these people do not usually attend clinic visits, they should be requested to attend at least one Stage 1 clinic visit. This allows relatives and caregivers to receive some training from the clinician.

Changing Treatment Structure During Stage 1. Early in Stage 1, when children's SRs often are high, treatment in structured conversations is arranged so that children's responses are mostly stutter-free. As they progress through Stage 1, their SRs decrease and treatment conversations become less structured. That is, clinician and parent adjust treatment structure as children increase the frequency and duration of their stutter-free responses. Consulting clinicians identified that incorrect adjustment of treatment structure was a contributing factor in 13% of consultations. Adjustment of treatment structure was found to be incorrect in one of two ways, in equal proportions: Either (1) structured treatment was used far too long, or (2) unstructured treatment was introduced far too early in Stage 1. In all cases, treatment was ineffective.

Suggestions

- In initial weeks of the Lidcombe Program, treatment occurs in structured conversations that ensure that there is much stutter-free speech. The other purpose of treatment in structured conversations is to ensure that the parent does it correctly and in a manner suitable for the child. Only then is treatment introduced into the unstructured conversations of daily life. Parents can use verbal contingencies for stutter-free and stuttered speech many times per day, in various conversations or situations. Although the parental contingencies are less frequent by then, the parent still maintains a 5:1 ratio of contingencies for stutter-free to stuttered speech.
- During each clinic visit, the parent and clinician consider changes to the treatment conducted at home. For this discussion to be well informed, the clinician collates various pieces of information. The parent is asked for details of treatment frequency, verbal contingencies, and child responses during treatment at home. The clinician gathers further information while observing the parent conduct treatment in the clinic. Then, the clinician guides subsequent discussion with the parent, during which they make decisions about treatment to be used in the week ahead.

Verbal Contingencies for Stutter-Free Speech. Problems with verbal contingencies occurred in 9% of consultations. One problem was that parents did not present enough contingencies for stutter-free speech. Their contingencies were presented either rarely or with the same frequency as their contingencies for stuttered speech.

Another problem with contingencies for stutter-free speech was that they were offered only in structured conversations but not in unstructured conversations. In each case, the children involved became unwilling to participate in treatment.

Suggestion

- Verbal contingencies for stutter-free speech need to be *at least* 5 times more frequent than contingencies for stuttered speech. It can be easy for parents, with the best of intentions, to change the focus of treatment onto the behavior they want to eliminate—stuttered speech—rather than the one they want to increase, which is stutter-free speech. Therefore, clinicians can check on the frequency of all aspects of treatment during their weekly discussions with parents during clinic visits.

Verbal Contingencies for Stuttered Speech. Incorrect use of contingencies for stuttered speech was identified as a contributing factor in 8% of consultations. There are several ways that contingencies for stuttering can be used incorrectly in the Lidcombe Program. Parents may present excessive contingencies for stuttering, or they may deliver them in ways that are unacceptable for children, or they may be inaccurate. In all cases, treatment is ineffective as children will either react negatively or simply ignore the contingencies.

Suggestions

- Children are sometimes particularly sensitive to their parent's manner of requesting self-corrections. One way to make them more acceptable is for the parent, using a quiet voice, to request the self-correction, and then continue the conversation as soon as the child responds. The exchange is brief and low-key, and the result is for self-corrections to become part of the conversational flow, and not highlighted in any way by the parent.
- The clinician can check accuracy of parental verbal contingencies for stuttered speech during clinic demonstrations of treatment by the parent, or by listening to audiotape recordings of treatment conducted elsewhere.

Treatment Frequency. In 8% of consultations, consulting clinicians identified low frequency of treatment in either structured or unstructured conversations as contributing to children's lack of progress in treatment. Complete absence of treatment outside clinic visits was one manifestation of this problem. More common was structured treatment being conducted by parents only once or twice each week.

Suggestions

- It is possible that clinicians may precipitate this problem by conducting all the treatment that occurs during clinic visits, leaving parents to be passive observers. If this occurs, then it may take some weeks to reorient parents to their new role of delivering daily treatment, gathering daily SRs, and consulting with the clinician during clinic visits.
- Treatment needs to occur every day throughout Stage 1. When structured treatment is used, it needs to occur at least once per day, and more often if necessary. When unstructured treatment is used, it needs to occur in several conversations each day.

Problems Related to Stage 2. Consulting clinicians found that problems relating to Stage 2 occurred in 5% of consultations. In a small number of cases, children had been placed in Stage 2 without achieving program speech criteria. When verbal contingencies were subsequently decreased, their SRs increased in frequency. In another case, problems arose after a child achieved speech criteria for Stage 2; however, parental verbal contingencies stopped completely in the first weeks of Stage 2, and the child's SRs increased.

Suggestions

- It can be helpful to remind parents during each of the early Stage 2 clinic visits about the need to withdraw verbal contingencies gradually. As gaps between clinic visits increase, parents can easily lose focus on the need to continue to monitor their children's speech and to be ready to respond immediately if stuttering increases.
- Every Stage 2 clinic visit is needed for discussion and consultation between parent and clinician. If a parent is unable to attend occasional clinic visits, then phone contact can be used instead, and taped samples of the child's speech can be mailed to the clinician.

Missing Components in Stage 1. In 5% of consultations, consulting clinicians concluded that a reason for the presenting problems was that clinicians were conducting treatment using only selected components of the Lidcombe Program. Advising speech pathologists identified that the most frequently missing components were weekly 1-hour clinic visits, parent training in the line of verbal contingencies, SRs, and consistent application of the treatment.

Suggestions

- Treatment outcome is unknown if only part of the Lidcombe Program is used, so all components should be included.
- It may be that a parent has difficulty with one component, such as remembering to collect an SR each day. Rather than leaving SRs out altogether, a far better solution is for the clinician and parent to discuss the problem and devise a solution that suits the parent.

Category 2: Parent and Child Issues that Affect Treatment

Child Has Other Speech–Language or Medical Problem. Consulting clinicians found that complications related to treatment of other problems were an issue in 8% of consultations. A factor identified as a possible reason for lack of progress in the Lidcombe Program was that clinicians were concurrently targeting several speech goals. Clinicians reported that they had clients with language, phonological, or dyspraxic difficulties as well as stuttering.

Suggestions

- Stuttering treatment is more effective when children are younger, and stuttering can become more severe over time. It therefore may be best to treat stuttering first, and initiate treatment for other disorders later, perhaps when the child is several months into Stage 2 (see Chapter 4).
- See Chapter 10 for discussion of special case studies.

Twins. An issue that arose in 2% of consultations concerned using the Lidcombe Program with twins who stuttered. Consulting clinicians noted that there were many difficulties in concurrently treating two young children. Clinicians asked for advice about issues such as whether to treat the children concurrently or consecutively, and what were reasonable expectations of treatment time.

Suggestions

- The clinician needs to discuss with the parent the particular household routines and organization. If the parent feels ready, the children can begin treatment at the same time, and if both children's SRs show improvement after a few weeks of Stage 1, continue the treatment.

- When the clinician starts treatment in the early Stage 1 clinic visits, it may be useful to treat the children separately. This allows the clinician and parent to determine optimal treatment for each child before attempting to conduct their treatments concurrently.

Sensitive Child. Aspects of the child's personality and age appeared as contributing problems in 2% of consultations. Clinicians reported children who were either sensitive about stuttering particularly, or generally sensitive about many things. A common characteristic among these children was that they were reported to dislike all verbal contingencies for their speech.

Suggestions

- Treatment can still be successful with sensitive children who react negatively to verbal contingencies. The parent learns to adjust the treatment in structured conversations so that the child's speech is consistently stutter-free and uses no verbal contingencies.
- Even with very sensitive children, it is often possible to introduce parental verbal contingencies, both for stutter-free and stuttered speech, part of the way through Stage 1. These contingencies can be introduced at a very low frequency, while the parent and clinician watch for any negative reaction from the child.
- It can be beneficial to decrease the directness of the request when asking a sensitive child to self-correct stuttered speech. For example:

  CHILD: Th-th-th-th-thaaaat one's mine.

  PARENT: (in a low-key manner) Can you say "that one's mine"?

  CHILD: That one's mine.

  PARENT: (more enthusiastically) Well done! You fixed that bumpy word.

  The parent did not mention the "bump" until *after* the child completed the self-correction. If the child was unable to correct the stutter, then the parent could acknowledge the attempt and continue the conversation.

- See Chapter 10 for discussion of special case studies.

Expectations of Treatment Outcome. In 2% of consultations, clinicians noted that treatment was affected by parents' skepticism about treatment outcome. One parent was reported to have requested a break from treatment due to feeling confused about how to proceed. Another parent was doubtful that treatment would be successful, as she herself had stuttered for many years despite having speech therapy. This parent felt that treatment might increase her child's stuttering. A third parent became discouraged because treatment duration was longer than expected.

Suggestions

- Give parents information about stuttering and the Lidcombe Program throughout Stage 1, starting at the first clinic visit. Initial information should be simple, with more detailed information made available as necessary.
- If it is considered necessary to give a parent a break from treatment, advise the parent to withdraw treatment at home. Otherwise, without ongoing advice and consultation with the clinician, treatment effectiveness probably will decline.

Problem Relationship Between Parent and Child. Problems encountered during 1% of consultations centered on difficult relationships between parent and child. In each case, parents focused consistently on their children's stuttering, without presenting contingencies for stutter-free speech.

Suggestions

- It can be helpful for the clinician to first explain to the parent that verbal contingencies are intended to be positive in tone. Then the clinician can demonstrate treatment, using only contingencies for stutter-free speech.
- In cases where the parent is unable to follow the clinician's model, the clinician can ask the parent to suggest acceptable verbal contingencies, and use these. That is, the clinician uses the parent's words. The child's response to these contingencies would be monitored in the usual manner.

Category 3: Child-Related Factors Not Directly Related to the Lidcombe Program

Stuttering Fluctuates. Advising clinicians found that 5% of consultations were initiated by concerns about fluctuating severity of children's stuttering. Clinicians reported that fluctuations were more pronounced when children were ill, upset, or excited.

In some cases, clinicians had not previously treated children whose stuttering varied greatly over days or weeks, and were not aware that this is common in early stuttering. In other cases, clinicians sought advice about how to measure treatment progress. The clinicians were aware that reductions in SRs may be due to treatment or to naturally occurring fluctuations. Consequently, they requested advice about how to direct treatment in these circumstances.

Suggestions

- There may not be any need to adjust treatment for children whose stuttering is characterized by large fluctuations in severity. As children progress through Stage 1, SR charts can be used to confirm progress over several weeks.
- Fluctuating SR patterns typically continue throughout Stage 1, with progress reflected in reduced range of SR fluctuations (see Figure 5.1).
- See Chapter 10 for discussion of special case studies.

Child Is Not Aware of Stuttering. A small portion of consultations (2%) concerned the children's lack of self-awareness of stuttering. Consulting clinicians requested advice about whether it was necessary, or wise, to make children aware of stuttering before starting the Lidcombe Program.

Suggestions

- It is not necessary for children to be aware of stuttering before starting the Lidcombe Program. Although their awareness typically increases during Stage 1, they are more likely to become aware of stutter-free speech, as it is the focus for more parental verbal contingencies than stuttered speech.
- It can be useful when parents ask children to self-evaluate their stutter-free speech.

Child Avoids Words. A single consultation was initiated by a clinician concerned about a child who avoided saying familiar words. During treatment sessions, the child occasionally would either substitute an incorrect word or leave a word out altogether. The clinician realized the implications of this if the child continued to avoid words, and sought advice on how to change treatment activities appropriately.

Suggestion

- Routine treatment will decrease stuttering and increase stutter-free speech, and the word substitutions and avoidance will disappear along the way. It is unlikely that any special treatment activities will be necessary.

Conclusion

The Lidcombe Program is used extensively by Australian speech pathologists who treat young stuttering children. Although most clinicians use the program without difficulty, there are times when advice will be needed from clinicians who have more experience using the program. For several years, Australian clinicians have had an opportunity to access such advice from the Stuttering Unit's phone consultation service. It has been routine practice in the unit to keep notes of each consultation for reference in case further consultation is requested on particular clients. Details of consultations regarding preschool-age children were gathered from the consulting clinicians during a series of interviews.

After analysis of the interview transcripts, it was found that there were two main reasons that consulting clinicians sought advice from the Stuttering Unit. First, two thirds of consultations were because preschool-age clients were not making progress in stuttering treatment. Second, the remaining one third of consultations were initiated by clinicians who identified gaps in their knowledge when working with relatively unusual clients. They sought advice about these issues, which were not directly related to the Lidcombe Program.

A second analysis of the consultation transcripts identified a wide range of issues that affected treatment. These issues were not the primary reasons for consultations, but were identified by advising clinicians as contributing to them. As such, this second analysis was a source of more detailed information about characteristics of preschool-age children, their families, stuttering, and the Lidcombe Program itself that may impede treatment progress and increase the likelihood that clinicians will request advice about treatment.

The information collected from our consultations confirms the need for comprehensive training for clinicians wanting to use the Lidcombe Program. Along with basic written information about the program, clinicians would benefit from learning about treating clients with issues that complicate their treatment, such as severe stuttering and sensitivity to verbal contingencies. Clinicians using the Lidcombe Program are also likely to benefit from advice from other clinicians more experienced in using the program. Examples of current advice sources for clinicians using the Lidcombe Program are the Stuttering Unit's telephone and e-mail consultation service,[1] the Lidcombe Link Days and the *Lidcombe News* in the United Kingdom (see Chapter 12), and *Lidcombe News Canada*.

[1] Information about the Stuttering Unit's consultation service is at http://www.swsahs.nsw.gov.au/stuttering

Part III

Case Studies

Chapter 9

Routine Case Studies

Isabelle Rousseau and Sue O'Brian

This chapter describes how the Lidcombe Program was used with 4 preschool-age children who stutter. The children differ in age, initial stuttering severity, personality, and family circumstances. However, there were no unusual factors that complicated their treatment. For each child, reasons for starting treatment and progression through the Lidcombe Program are outlined. The charts of clinical measures for each child, showing their progress through Stage 1 of the program, are provided. The children's names have been altered.

Oliver

Assessment

Oliver was age 4 years 9 months when his mother brought him to our clinic for assessment of stuttering and advice about treatment. The onset of his stuttering was sudden, and had occurred 10 months earlier. Since then, his stuttering severity had fluctuated between mild and severe. Referral to our clinic was prompted by an extended period of particularly severe stuttering a few weeks earlier.

Ms. B (Oliver's mother) was very concerned about Oliver's stuttering because her brother stuttered severely. She had noticed that Oliver's awareness of his stuttering had increased recently. She reported that he put his hand over his mouth when he stuttered and on one occasion had grabbed his mouth, apparently in frustration. She described Oliver's stutters as consisting mainly of repeated syllables and words. She reported that she had been reluctant to do or say anything to help him because she thought Oliver was already sensitive about his stuttering.

During the clinic visit, Oliver seemed to be shy and was reluctant to talk with either the clinician or his mother. An audiotaped speech sample, recorded at home and brought to the assessment, was therefore used to obtain a measure of percentage of syllables stuttered (%SS). Stuttering rate was 12%SS, and Oliver's stutters were primarily syllable repetitions and some fixed postures with audible airflow. "Fixed postures with audible airflow" are also referred to as "prolongation" or "sound prolongation."

The clinician recommended that Oliver start the Lidcombe Program, and his mother agreed. This recommendation was made for these reasons:

- It was 10 months since onset of his stuttering.
- His stuttering was causing him frustration.
- His stuttering showed no signs of decreasing in severity.
- He was due to start school in 4 months.

The clinician demonstrated to Ms. B how to conduct treatment in a structured conversation. Oliver was enjoying playing with farm animals at the time, so these were used during the demonstrations. Ms. B then conducted treatment, and Oliver was able to produce one- and two-word responses that were consistently stutter-free. She acknowledged and praised his stutter-free responses, and he increased the length of his stutter-free utterances to three- and four-word phrases.

Before the end of the clinic visit, the clinician summarized what Ms. B was to do during the week ahead:

- Ms. B would collect two severity ratings (SRs) each day and record them on a chart (see Figure 9.1). These SRs would reflect Oliver's least severe and most severe stuttering. Figure 9.1 presents the more severe SRs each day.
- Ms. B would audiotape one 10-minute sample of Oliver's speech in conversation.
- Ms. B and Oliver would do a 10-minute structured treatment each day, as demonstrated during the clinic visit.

Stage 1

Clinic Visit 1

▶ Within-Clinic Speech Measure: 7%SS

The clinician and Ms. B listened to a speech sample recorded at home and identified each stutter. At first, Ms. B did not recognize that Oliver's fixed postures with audible airflow were stutters. Following instruction from the clinician, she was able to do this successfully.

Ms. B reported that Oliver had enjoyed treatment in structured conversations at home, and that they had conducted treatment for approximately 5 minutes each day. Ms. B then demonstrated treatment, and Oliver's responses were consistently stutter-free phrases and short sentences. Ms. B used a variety of verbal contingencies following stutter-free speech, but these referred to Oliver (e.g., "Good boy!") rather than to his stutter-free speech. The clinician and Ms. B discussed more appropriate contingencies to use during the week ahead.

The clinician and Ms. B then discussed how to introduce verbal contingencies for Oliver's stuttered speech. They agreed that Ms. B would only acknowledge his stutters and would not request self-corrections. If Oliver accepted these contingencies, then requests for self-correction would be introduced later.

Ms. B continued the structured treatment, using contingencies for both stutter-free and stuttered speech. Oliver enjoyed the activities, which continued for nearly 20 minutes. The clinician therefore asked Ms. B to increase the time spent in structured conversations at home.

Clinic Visit 2

▶ Within-Clinic Speech Measure: 5%SS

The clinician again checked the reliability of Ms. B's SRs. Ms. B confirmed that Oliver's speech sample in the clinic was typical of his speech at home during the previous week.

Ms. B demonstrated treatment in structured conversations with Oliver and confirmed that he still enjoyed doing these treatments each day. She reported that his responses were short sentences that were consistently stutter-free. The main change to treatment made during this clinic visit was to introduce requests for Oliver to self-correct stutters occasionally. Initially, Ms. B was reluctant to do this, as she was unsure of Oliver's reaction. The clinician demonstrated treatment and used verbal contingencies for stutter-free and stuttered speech, and Oliver continued to enjoy the activity as before. The clinician emphasized that Ms. B should not ask Oliver to self-correct more than two stutters per structured treatment, and al-

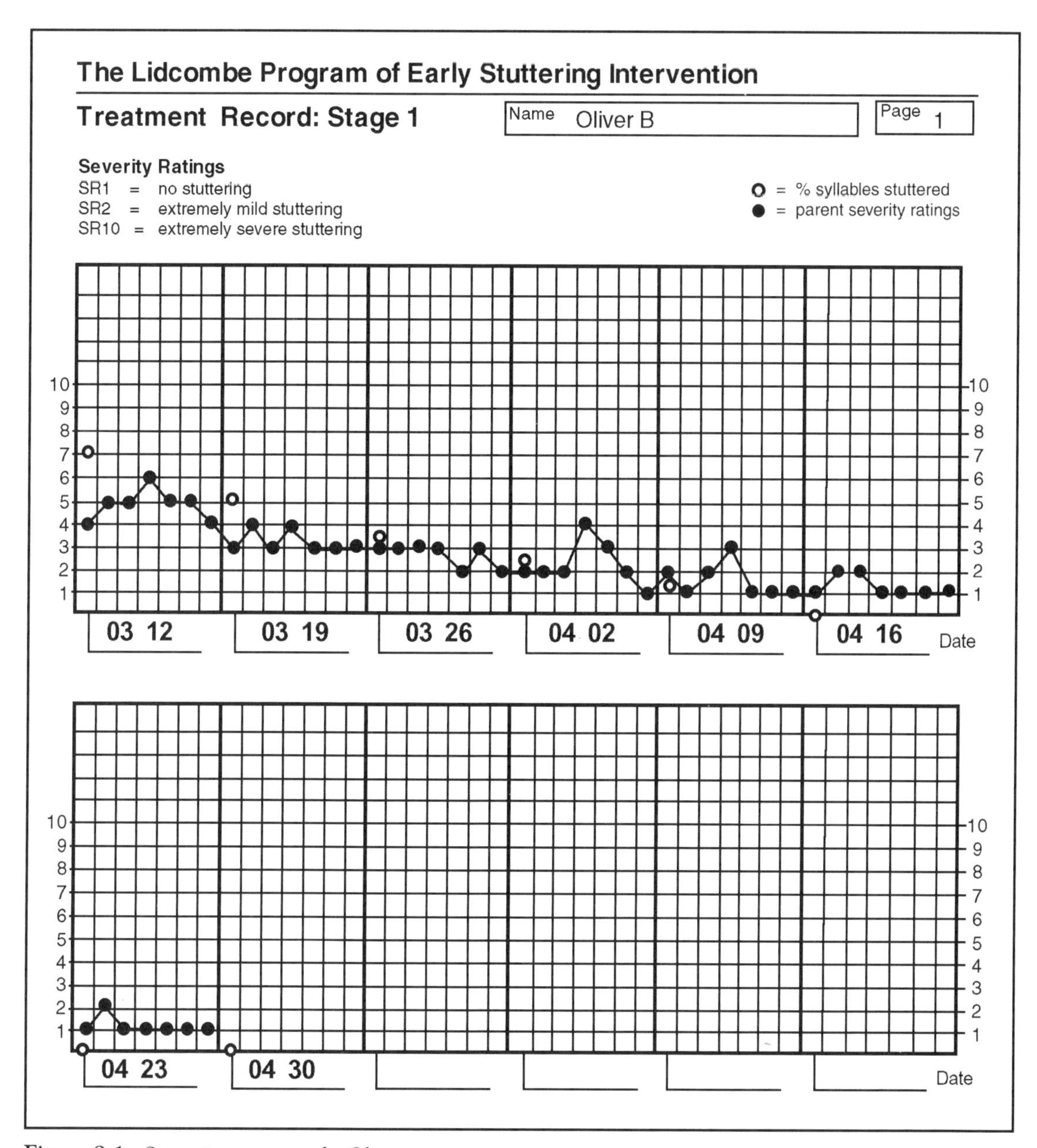

Figure 9.1. Stuttering measures for Oliver.

ways to do so in conjunction with frequent praise for stutter-free speech.

Clinic Visit 3

▶ Within-Clinic Speech Measure: 3.5%SS

Ms. B reported a general decrease in Oliver's stuttering during the previous week. She noted that his highest severity rating was 4, he was virtually always stutter-free during treatment in structured conversation, and he had spontaneously self-corrected some stuttered speech during conversation. These observations led the clinician to recommend two changes in treatment: (1) that Ms. B praise Oliver for spontaneously self-correcting stutters and (2) that she present verbal contingencies for Oliver's stutter-free and stuttered speech in unstructured conversations. The clinician suggested that, following a treatment in structured conversation, Ms. B could prompt Oliver to continue using stutter-free speech during everyday speech. This could occur while they, for example, walked to the park or played a game together.

Clinic Visit 4

▶ **Within-Clinic Speech Measure: 2.5%SS**

A significant change recommended was that Ms. B reduce the frequency of treatment in structured conversations to four per week. The clinician recommended that treatment continue to occur each day in unstructured conversations, with Ms. B using verbal contingencies for stutter-free and stuttered speech.

Clinic Visit 5

▶ **Within-Clinic Speech Measure: 1.5%SS**

Ms. B reported that Oliver had an SR of 4 during his sister's birthday party, when he was extremely excited. Ms. B reported that she did a structured treatment with him on the following day, and his SR had decreased again immediately. The clinician confirmed that Ms. B had responded appropriately to Oliver's increased SR.

The clinician and Ms. B agreed that Oliver's treatment for the week ahead should be solely in unstructured conversations, and that structured treatment would be used only if his SR was 4 or higher.

Clinic Visit 6

▶ **Within-Clinic Speech Measure: 0%SS**

Ms. B commented that she had inadvertently reduced the frequency of her verbal contingencies for Oliver's stutter-free speech. Because his stutters were infrequent, she had forgotten to do treatment. On a day that he had an SR of 3, Oliver's increased stuttering prompted her to think about his speech again, and she realized that they had not done any treatment for the past 3 days. She immediately started to acknowledge and praise his stutter-free speech in unstructured conversations. The clinician reinforced that her response to Oliver's SR of 3 was correct.

The clinician asked for an estimate of the number of verbal contingencies used each day. Ms. B reported using verbal contingencies for stutter-free speech 20 to 25 times, and for stuttered speech 5 to 8 times per day. The clinician recommended that Ms. B continue treatment in the same manner for the week ahead.

Clinic Visit 7

▶ **Within-Clinic Speech Measure: 0%SS**

The clinician described Stage 2 of the Lidcombe Program to Ms. B, including the speech criteria for entering it. As well as continuing to collect daily SRs, the clinician asked Ms. B to listen to one 10-minute sample of Oliver's speech each week, and to count the number of stutters in each sample.

Clinic Visit 8

▶ **Within-Clinic Speech Measure: 0%SS**

After hearing Ms. B's report that she heard no stutters during the 10-minute samples during the week, the clinician confirmed that Oliver was ready to start Stage 2. She recommended that Ms. B continue her current treatment routine, that is, verbal contingencies during unstructured conversations for both stutter-free and stuttered speech, until Oliver's first Stage 2 clinic visit in 2 weeks.

Stage 2

The standard speech criteria and schedule for the program were used (see Chapter 7):

- Severity ratings (SRs) for each day of the week are 1 or 2, with at least four of these being 1.
- Percentage of syllables stuttered (%SS) within the clinic is below 1.0.

Oliver completed Stage 2 uneventfully, in the scheduled time frame. He was discharged 44 weeks later.

Lucy

Assessment

Lucy was age 3 years 8 months when she was assessed. Onset of stuttering had occurred suddenly 8 months earlier. An episode of severe stuttering, which lasted several weeks, had occurred shortly after that. During that episode, Lucy became very frustrated with her stuttering, and her parents said that they could barely understand her. By the time of her assessment, the severity of Lucy's stuttering had decreased a little and her speech was intelligible.

Lucy's stuttering rate during a conversation in the clinic was 10%SS. Her stutters consisted mainly of repetition of syllables and words and a few fixed postures. Her parents reported this was typical of Lucy's stuttering at home, although they occasionally saw her blinking while she stuttered. Stuttering rate for a second sample of Lucy's speech, recorded at home, was 7%SS. Lucy seemed to have no negative reactions to her stuttering, although her parents were sure that she was aware of it. There was no reported family history of stuttering. Following this assessment, Lucy's name was placed on the waiting list for treatment, and her name reached the top of the waiting list 7 months later.

Stage 1

Clinic Visit 1

▶ Within-Clinic Speech Measure: 8%SS

Lucy's stuttering consisted of frequent syllable repetitions, with up to eight iterations per stutter, and occasional fixed postures with audible airflow. Ms. M (Lucy's mother) said that this sample was typical of Lucy's speech at home.

As the severity of Lucy's stuttering was stable across each day, the clinician asked Ms. M to chart one SR per day. The clinician and Ms. M then listened to a taped sample of Lucy's speech and identified each stutter as it occurred. Ms. M was consistently accurate in identifying stutters. No treatment was trialed due to time constraints. Stuttering measures for Lucy are shown in Figure 9.2.

Clinic Visit 2

▶ Within-Clinic Speech Measure: 8%SS

Ms. M had no difficulty making SRs. Lucy's speech sample in the clinic was again apparently typical of her speech at home.

The clinician demonstrated structured treatment, using books as stimulus material. Contingencies for stutter-free speech were token rewards, acknowledgment, and various forms of praise. The conversation was structured so that Lucy was able to say short sentences that were consistently stutter-free. Ms. M watched the clinician's demonstration for a few minutes and then continued the treatment with Lucy, during which Lucy started to talk more spontaneously, and to stutter. The clinician prompted Ms. M to introduce more structure to the conversation, and Lucy's responses became shorter and stutter-free. The clinician reinforced that this was the type of structured conversation to use for treatment in the week ahead. She recommended that Ms. M and Lucy spend

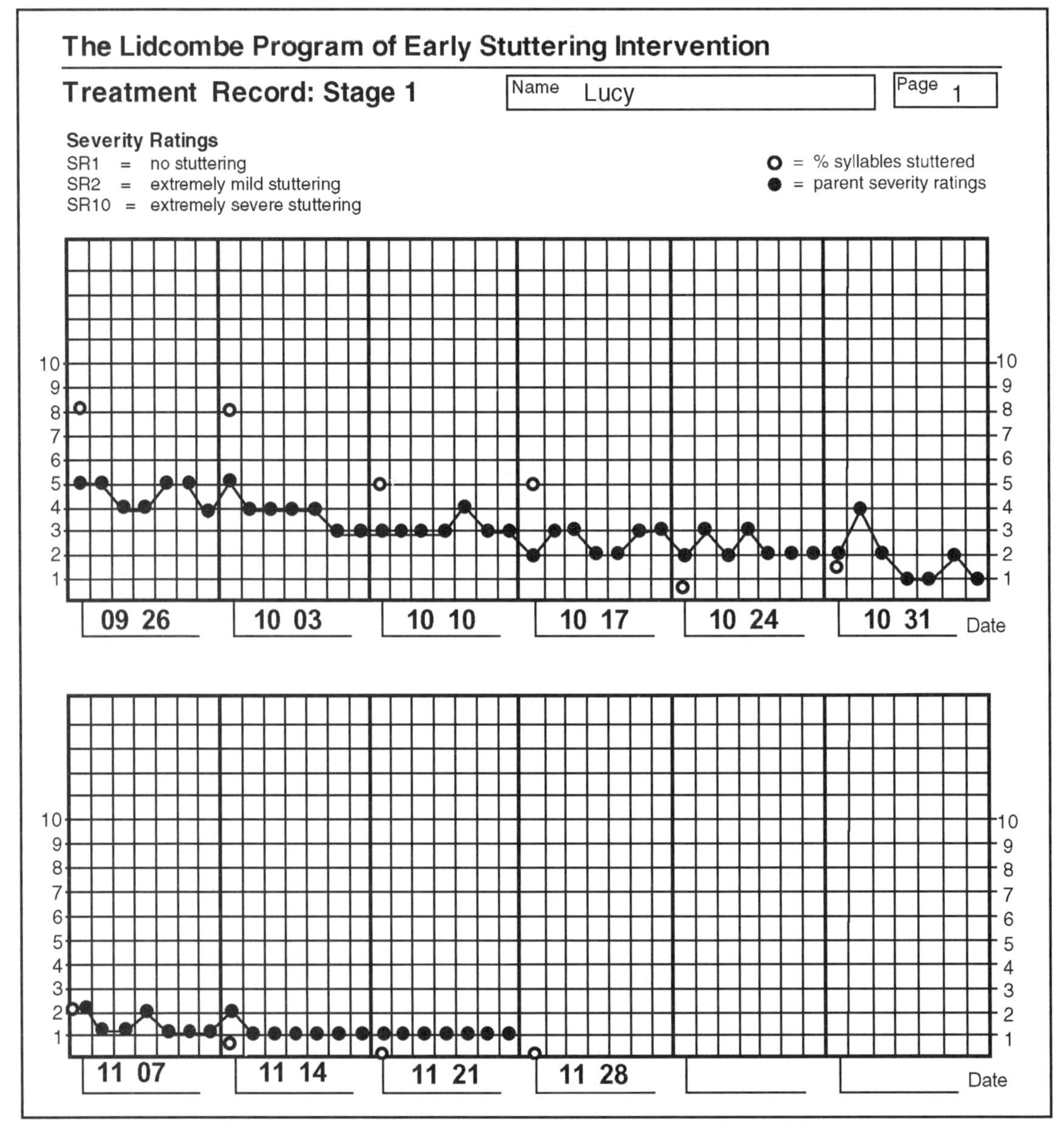

Figure 9.2. Stuttering measures for Lucy.

10 minutes each morning doing treatment in this format.

Clinic Visit 3

▶ Within-Clinic Speech Measure: 6%SS

Ms. M reported that she and Lucy had completed at least one structured treatment, and sometimes two, each day, usually at lunchtime. Lucy enjoyed these, and was consistently stutter-free while saying short sentences. Ms. M briefly demonstrated treatment with Lucy, and the clinician confirmed that it was being done correctly. The clinician then explained and demonstrated contingencies for stuttered speech during unstructured conversations.

For the following week, Ms. M agreed to do structured treatment every day, using contingencies for stutter-free and stuttered speech. She also agreed to start using contingencies for stutter-free speech during unstructured conversations.

Clinic Visit 4

▶ Within-Clinic Speech Measure: 5%SS

Therapy consisted of structured treatment for 10 minutes each day, as well as treatment during unstructured conversations. Ms. M reported using toys and puzzles during structured treatment, as Lucy preferred these to books.

The clinician recommended that Ms. M decrease the frequency of structured treatment, and increase treatment during unstructured conversations. They agreed that Ms. M would not do structured treatment on the days that Lucy attended preschool.

Clinic Visit 5

▶ Within-Clinic Speech Measure: 0.5%SS

Ms. M reported that she had tended to forget to do unstructured treatment. She felt that this was due to the reduction in Lucy's stuttering; that is, she was prompted to do treatment by Lucy's stutters rather than her stutter-free speech. Ms. M also said that she found it hard to distinguish between stuttering and normal word repetitions. The clinician advised her to respond to unambiguous stuttering only.

The clinician recommended that Ms. M continue unstructured treatment each day and decrease the amount of structured treatment. The clinician requested that she tape-record a 10-minute sample of Lucy's speech at home and bring it to the next clinic visit.

Clinic Visit 6

▶ Within-Clinic Speech Measure:1.5%SS

Ms. M reported that Lucy's stutters were all repetitions, with two to three iterations per stutter. Relatives and neighbors had noticed the improvement in Lucy's speech.

Unstructured treatment occurred each day in conversations. Ms. M reported using verbal contingencies for stuttering four or five times per day, and contingencies for stutter-free speech 25 to 30 times per day.

Clinic Visit 7

▶ Within-Clinic Speech Measure: 2%SS

Ms. M reported that Lucy had suddenly stuttered much more one day, but could not recall any circumstance that may have been related to this. She had increased the frequency of her verbal contingencies on that day, and all treatment was conducted in unstructured conversations. The clinician reinforced Ms. M's decision to adjust treatment in response to Lucy's SR. On a tape recording of Lucy's speech, Ms. M and the clinician agreed on an SR of 2.

The clinician asked Ms. M to try to count Lucy's stutters on one day during the forthcoming week. She also asked Ms. M to obtain a stopwatch to use for measuring stutters per minute of speaking time (SMST) at the next clinic visit.

Clinic Visit 8

▶ Within-Clinic Speech Measure: 0.5%SS

The clinician recommended that Ms. M continue frequent verbal contingencies for stutter-free speech during unstructured conversations, and to ask Lucy to self-correct each stutter.

During SMST training, Ms. M initially counted each of Lucy's normally disfluent repeated words and brief pauses as stutters. She became more accurate after discussion with the clinician about stutters and normal speech in preschool-age children. The SMST score for the tape was 0.7.

Clinic Visit 9

▶ Within-Clinic Speech Measure: 0%SS

Treatment had continued in unstructured conversations, and Lucy had self-corrected each stutter when requested. Lucy had also spontaneously started to self-correct stutters, and to comment on how smoothly she was talking. The clinician recommended that Ms. M praise these responses, as well as Lucy's stutter-free speech.

SMST scores for two tapes were 0.7 and 0. The clinician told Ms. M that it was likely that Lucy would progress to Stage 2 after her next clinic visit.

Clinic Visit 10

▶ Within-Clinic Speech Measure: 0%SS

Lucy met criteria for Stage 2 (SMST score was 0). The clinician recommended that Ms. M make no changes to treatment until the first Stage 2 clinic visit.

Stage 2

Lucy passed through Stage 2, with standard speech criteria and standard schedule (see Chapter 7), without failing to meet program speech criteria. Her parents noted no stutters after the second clinic visit. Lucy was discharged 10 months later.

Bill

Assessment

Bill was age 4 years 1 month at the time of assessment and had been stuttering for around 18 months. Onset had been gradual, but the severity of his stuttering had been consistent for the past 14 months. Ms. J (Bill's mother) had been concerned about Bill's stuttering for some time, but his preschool teacher had assured her that he would grow out of it, so Ms. J had delayed referring Bill for assessment.

Ms. J had tried to help Bill by getting him to slow his speech and start again after each stutter. Although he usually could then repeat these utterances without stuttering, Ms. J felt it made no overall effect on his stuttering severity.

There was no history of stuttering in Bill's immediate family. His cousin stuttered for a short time but had recovered without clinical intervention.

At his assessment, Bill presented as an outgoing, friendly, and cooperative boy. In conversation, stuttering rate was 5%SS and severity was SR 5. His stutters were mainly syllable repetitions. His parents described this sample as less severe than his typical stuttering, which commonly included fixed postures with audible airflow.

The clinician recommended that Bill start the Lidcombe Program for the following reasons:

- Significant and persistent stuttering
- 18 months since onset
- Stuttering was not decreasing since onset
- Bill was to begin school in 6 months

Treatment started 4 months later.

Stage 1

Clinic Visit 1

▶ Within-Clinic Speech Measure: 15%SS

Ms. J described Bill's clinic speech sample as typical of his least severe stuttering during previous weeks. She noticed that his stuttering severity varied according to his level of excitement and tiredness. The clinician therefore suggested that Ms. J collect an SR for 10 minutes of Bill's speech in conversation per day, and sample several situations across the week. They discussed Bill's weekly routine, and agreed on these situations: bath time (Mondays, Thursdays), walking home from preschool (Tuesdays, Wednesdays), playing with his brother (Fridays, Sundays), and gardening with Dad (Saturdays). Stuttering measures for Bill are shown in Figure 9.3.

The clinician introduced treatment in structured conversations to Bill with a simple explanation and then demonstrated how this could be done looking at a storybook. At the beginning of the activity, Bill gave one- and two-word responses, and the clinician's verbal contingencies were for stutter-free speech. After a few minutes, Bill was enjoying the activity, and his speech was consistently stutter-free. The clinician adjusted the structure of the conversation so that Bill's responses were either phrases or short sentences. Contingencies for stuttered speech were then introduced, and Bill was able to self-correct each stutter. The clinician asked Ms. J to attempt treatment in the structured conversation, and after taking a while to familiarize herself with the procedure, she continued treatment in the same manner as the clinician.

To conclude the clinic visit, the clinician and Ms. J discussed the speech measures and treatment that would be done during the following week.

Clinic Visit 2

▶ **Within-Clinic Speech Measure: 15%SS**

Ms. J reported that she had not collected SRs in the manner discussed at the previous clinic visit. She forgot to listen closely to Bill's speech in the selected situations on the first 2 days of the week. Subsequently, she collected one overall SR for each day and found that this was easier to do.

Ms. J said that, although she had felt very apprehensive about conducting treatment, once she had "given it a go," she found that Bill enjoyed treatment in structured conversation and she found it satisfying to help him. She demonstrated the procedure, and the clinician suggested that Ms. J increase the duration of Bill's stutter-free responses before providing a verbal contingency.

Clinic Visit 3

▶ **Within-Clinic Speech Measure: 6%SS**

Ms. J reported that several friends had noticed the reduction in Bill's stuttering, which also was reflected in his SRs. His stutters were syllable repetitions and occasional fixed postures with audible airflow. She also reported feeling reasonably confident about the way she was doing the structured treatment. She also reported that Bill enjoyed treatment and reminded her if she forgot to do a "speech game" with him after breakfast.

Ms. J and Bill demonstrated treatment in a structured conversation. During this demon-stration, Bill spontaneously self-corrected some stutters, and the clinician recommended that Ms. J praise these responses.

The clinician and Ms. J discussed treatment in the week ahead. They agreed that treatment would continue each day, in unstructured conversations when Bill's SR was 3 or lower, and in structured conversations if his SR was higher.

Clinic Visit 4

▶ **Within-Clinic Speech Measure: 5%SS**

Ms. J confirmed that treatment continued successfully. The clinician confirmed that her SRs were reliable, and that Bill was still enjoying treatment. The clinician instructed Ms. J to increase the number of verbal contingencies during treatment in unstructured conversations.

Clinic Visit 5

▶ **Within-Clinic Speech Measure: 8%SS**

Bill was ill during the previous week and refused to do the treatment on 4 consecutive days. Ms. J was concerned about his increased SRs that resulted from this, but realized that it would be counterproductive to attempt treatment when he was unwilling to do it. The clinician confirmed that Bill's decreased

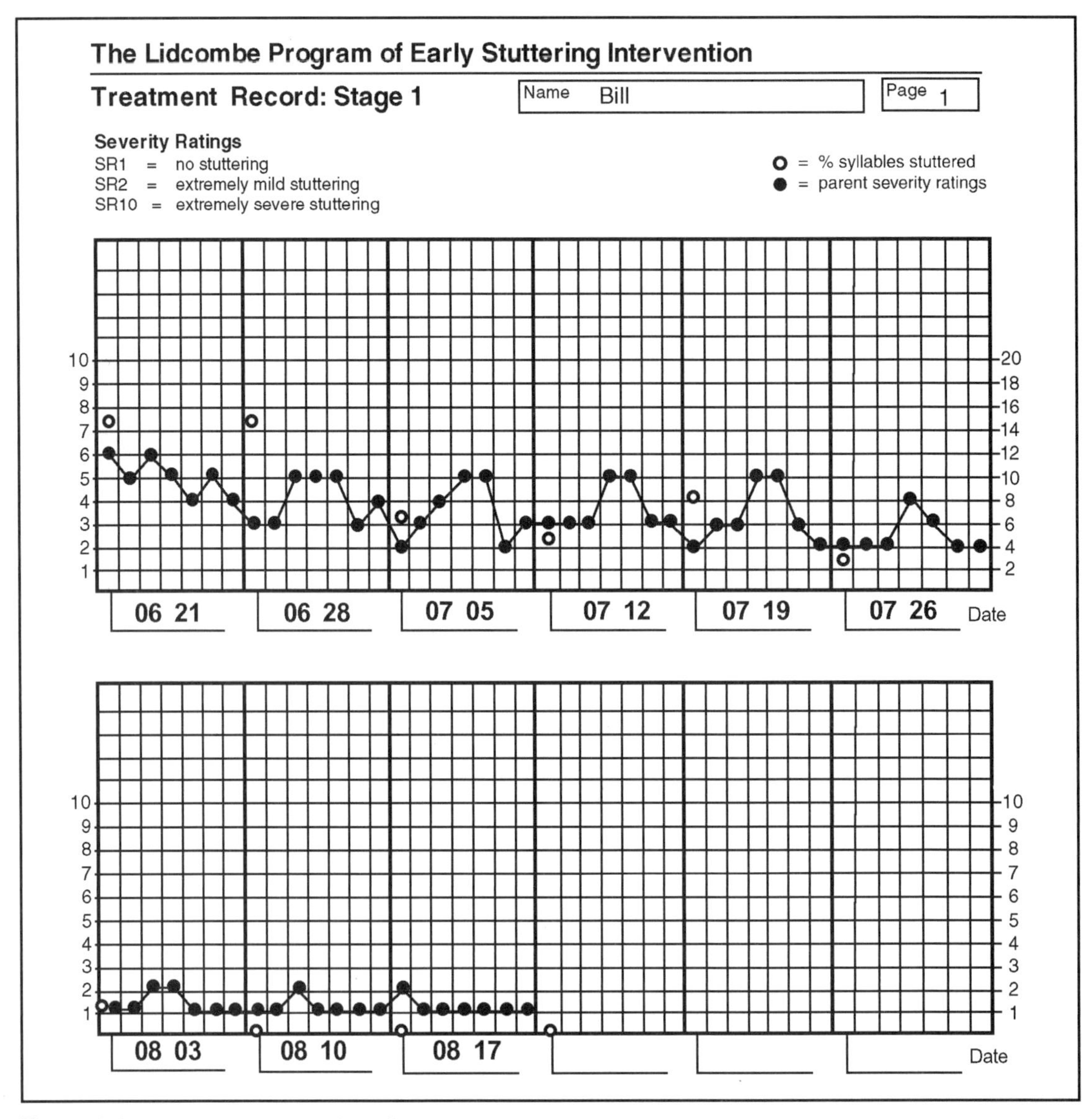

Figure 9.3. Stuttering measures for Bill.

SRs at the end of the week suggested that she had made a good decision.

Clinic Visit 6

▶ Within-Clinic Speech Measure: 3%SS

Ms. J commented that Bill always had an SR of 1 during treatment in structured conversations, and then his stuttering would increase gradually over the next hour. The clinician discussed with her how treatment could occur during many routine unstructured conversations, for example, while walking to the park or while baking a cake together.

Clinic Visit 7

▶ Within-Clinic Speech Measure: 2%SS

Stuttering measures showed a pattern of low SRs on weekdays and higher SRs on weekends.

Ms. J attributed this to high levels of noise, activity, excitement, and arguing that occurred when Bill and his three siblings were together for long periods. The clinician advised Ms. J to do treatment in structured conversations as early as possible on Saturdays and Sundays, and then to continue verbal contingencies for stutter-free speech in unstructured conversations later in the day. The clinician also discussed with Ms. J how she could use SRs to monitor Bill's response to treatment over the weekend.

Clinic Visit 8

▶ **Within-Clinic Speech Measure: 0%SS**

Most of the clinic visit was spent discussing details of therapy, including the amount of structured and unstructured treatment during the previous week. The clinician recommended that Bill's treatment in the week ahead should be in unstructured conversations only, with verbal contingencies for stutter-free and stuttered speech. She recommended that structured treatment be used only if Bill's SRs went to 3 or higher.

Clinic Visit 9

▶ **Within-Clinic Speech Measure: 0%SS**

The clinician confirmed that Bill was likely to finish Stage 1 in a week. She briefly described to Ms. J the Stage 2 speech criteria and the schedule of clinic visits during Stage 2. She also asked Ms. J to record a 10-minute speech sample to be used to measure SMST at the next visit.

Clinic Visit 10

▶ **Within-Clinic Speech Measure: 0%SS**

Ms. J reported that she had heard only three stutters during the previous week. Bill's SRs were supplemented by a 10-minute sample of him talking with his grandmother. The clinician and Ms. J measured this sample as 0.4 SMST. The clinician confirmed that Bill would now progress to Stage 2. She recommended that Ms. J continue treatment until Bill's first Stage 2 clinic visit. The clinician recommended that Ms. J focus on not forgetting to acknowledge Bill's stutter-free speech.

Stage 2

Standard speech criteria and a standard schedule (see Chapter 7) were used. Bill progressed uneventfully through Stage 2. Ms. J gradually withdrew verbal contingencies over the first 8 weeks of Stage 2 and Bill was discharged 10 months later.

Dean

Assessment

Dean was age 3 years 4 months at the time of assessment. Reportedly he began to stutter when he was just older than 2 years old. His parents said that the onset of his stuttering was sudden, and his stutters at first were repetitions and prolongations. Over the next few months, his stuttering frequency increased and the type of stuttering changed. At the time of his assessment, prolongations and blocks were his most common types of stuttering. A sample of Dean's speech in a conversation during the clinic visit showed 18%SS, and his parents said that this was typical of his speech in the preceding weeks. Mr. and Ms. L (Dean's parents) reported that Dean was acutely aware of his stuttered speech and had at times reacted negatively. They recalled one incident that occurred a month earlier: Dean's sister had talked for him while he was stuttering on a long narrative. Dean had thrown himself on the floor and yelled at his sister to "stop talking." On other occasions, he commented, "I can't get the words out" or "I make bad words." There was a history of stuttering among Dean's relatives: His father, paternal grandfather, and a maternal aunt stuttered.

Dean's name was placed on the waiting list, and 5 months later he started the Lidcombe Program, at age 4 years 0 months. Stuttering measures for Dean are shown in Figure 9.4.

Stage 1

Clinic Visit 1

▶ Within-Clinic Speech Measure: 12%SS

Ms. L reported that there had been little change in the severity or frequency of Dean's stuttered speech since his initial assessment 5 months earlier. The clinician explained severity ratings to Ms. L and asked her to assign a rating to Dean's speech while they talked and played with toys for 10 minutes. Ms. L assigned an SR of 6, and further discussion revealed that this was typical of Dean's speech in recent weeks. The clinician and Ms. L discussed various means of collecting SRs, and agreed that Ms. L would collect one SR per day for the entire day.

The clinician demonstrated treatment in structured conversations, using only verbal contingencies for stutter-free speech and giving him parts of a building set contingent on each of Dean's stutter-free responses. He was consistently stutter-free while saying three- or four-word phrases, but he stuttered on longer utterances. When Ms. L attempted to do the same treatment with him, Dean refused to cooperate. The clinician recommended that Ms. L collect and chart an SR each day during the week ahead, but not start treatment. She also recommended that Ms. L think about books and games that would be suitable for Dean and bring one or two of Dean's favorite books to the next clinic visit.

Clinic Visit 2

▶ Within-Clinic Speech Measure: 14%SS

Ms. L brought to the clinic two of Dean's favorite books. After discussion about Dean's SRs in the clinic and at home during the previous week, the clinician demonstrated structured treatment for a short period. Ms. L then continued the same activity with Dean, giving him parts of a toy set and acknowledgment and praise for each stutter-free response, most of which were short phrases. Dean stuttered occasionally, but no verbal contingencies were applied to these.

The clinician and Ms. L discussed treatment for the week ahead, and Ms. L agreed that she and Dean would do 10 to 15 minutes of structured treatment each morning. Ms. L would acknowledge and praise his stutter-free speech during structured treatments and also in unstructured conversations. However, the clinician reminded Ms. L that most of Dean's speech in unstructured conversations would be stuttered. They agreed that no verbal contingencies would be applied to Dean's stuttered speech in either structured or unstructured treatments.

Clinic Visit 3

▶ Within-Clinic Speech Measure: 12%SS

Ms. L reported that several relatives had been staying with them during the previous week for a family celebration. Due to these circumstances, she and Dean had been unable to do many structured treatments during the previous week.

Ms. L and the clinician discussed treatment for the week ahead. Ms. L expected that family routines would be back to normal, and that structured treatments would therefore occur each day.

Clinic Visit 4

▶ Within-Clinic Speech Measure: 10%SS

Ms. L reported that Dean had been ill during the week, and his SR was highest on days when

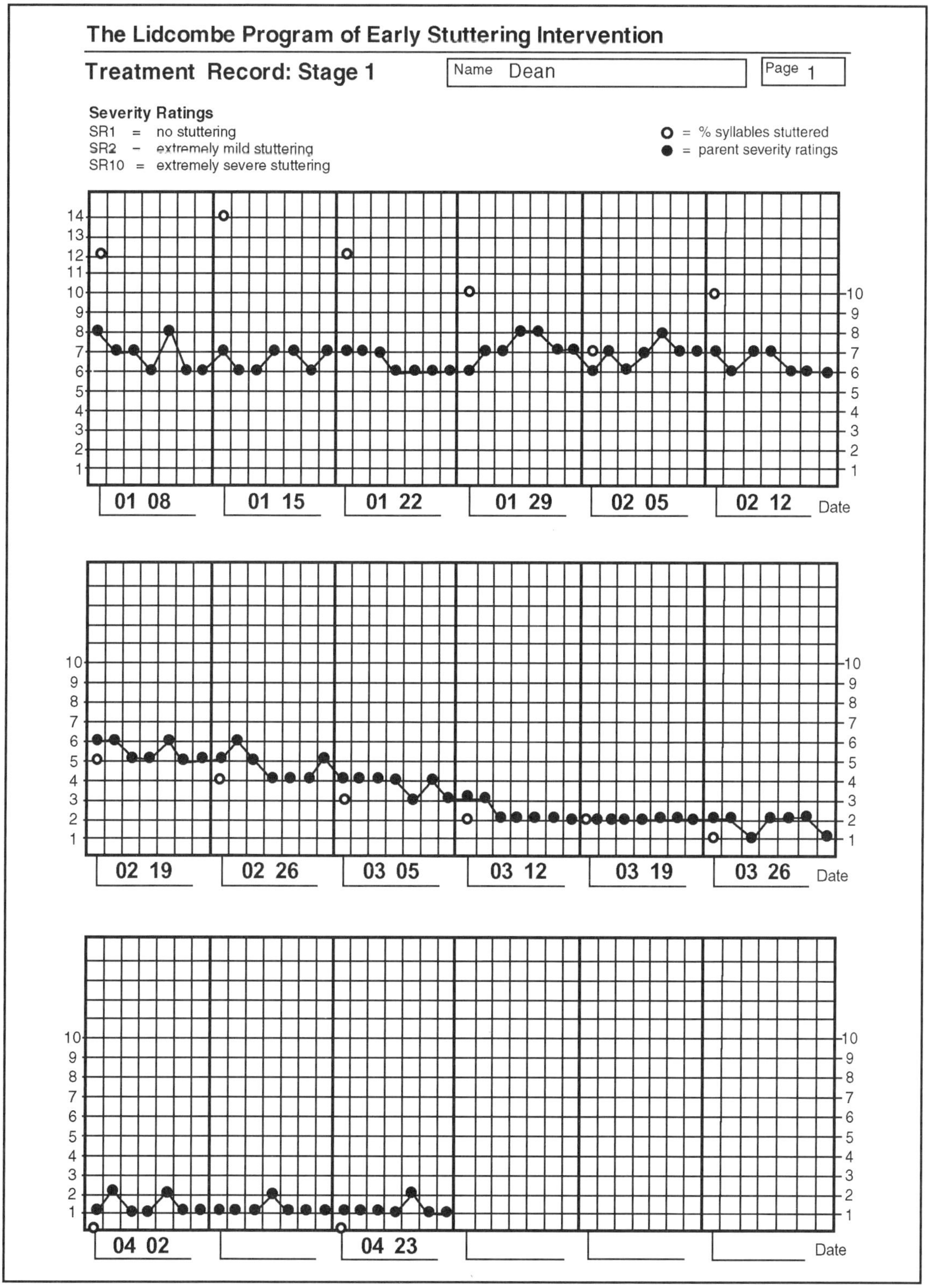

The Lidcombe Program of Early Stuttering Intervention

Treatment Record: Stage 1

Name Dean

Page 1

Severity Ratings

SR1 = no stuttering
SR2 = extremely mild stuttering
SR10 = extremely severe stuttering

O = % syllables stuttered
● = parent severity ratings

01 08 | 01 15 | 01 22 | 01 29 | 02 05 | 02 12 Date

02 19 | 02 26 | 03 05 | 03 12 | 03 19 | 03 26 Date

04 02 | | 04 23 | | | Date

Figure 9.4. Stuttering measures for Dean.

he was ill. She reported doing at least one, and sometimes two, structured treatments each day. Dean enjoyed these treatments, and Ms. L reported that he was consistently stutter-free while saying three- or four-word utterances. Dean stuttered no more than four times per structured treatment, and Ms. L had not asked Dean to self-correct these.

When demonstrating treatment during the clinic visit, Ms. L elicited four- to five-word stutter-free utterances. After a few minutes, the clinician described to Ms. L how to use verbal contingencies for stuttered speech and asked her to include these as she continued. Over the next 10 minutes of treatment in structured conversations, Dean produced longer utterances, most of which were stutter-free.

The clinician recommended that Ms. L continue daily treatment in structured conversations using contingencies for stutter-free and stuttered speech. She also recommended that Ms. L use contingencies for stutter-free utterances in unstructured conversations.

Clinic Visit 5

▶ Within-Clinic Speech Measure: 7%SS

Ms. L reported that both Dean and she were ill during the previous week. Nevertheless, other people had commented to her on how his speech had improved. Treatment in structured conversations had been conducted on most days, except for one day when Ms. L was ill.

Ms. L's demonstration of structured treatment showed that Dean was consistently stutter-free while saying five- to six-word utterances. The clinician suggested allowing Dean to say longer utterances. Dean stuttered a little more and Ms. L adjusted the activity to ensure that most of his responses were stutter-free.

Ms. L agreed to continue treatment at home, and to adjust the structured conversations as necessary to ensure Dean's speech was mostly stutter-free.

Clinic Visit 6

▶ Within-Clinic Speech Measure: 10%SS

Dean attended the clinic visit with his father, as Ms. L was unable to attend. Mr. L did not bring Dean's SR chart and was unable to report details of treatment conducted at home. The clinic visit therefore was short, and the clinician recommended that Ms. L continue treatment without changes for the time being.

Clinic Visit 7

▶ Within-Clinic Speech Measure: 5%SS

Ms. L reported that Dean's stuttering had been more stable during the past week than the previous week, and that friends had commented on the improvement in his speech. Structured and unstructured treatment occurred each day, with structured treatment for 10 minutes each morning and acknowledge and praise for stutter-free speech during unstructured conversations at various times each day.

Ms. L demonstrated her treatment in unstructured conversations, giving Dean frequent praise for his stutter-free utterances and occasionally requesting him to self-correct stutters. Dean spontaneously self-corrected several times, and Ms. L praised each of these responses. The clinician and Ms. L agreed that unstructured treatment in the week ahead would include verbal contingencies for Dean's stutter-free and stuttered speech, and for his spontaneous self-corrections.

Clinic Visit 8

▶ Within-Clinic Speech Measure: 4%SS

Ms. L reported further improvement in Dean's speech during the previous week. Structured and unstructured treatment continued each day, and Ms. L reported that she had praised Dean's spontaneous self-corrections on several occasions. Ms. L demonstrated unstructured treatment during the clinic visit, and the clinician recommended that she increase the frequency of her verbal contingencies for Dean's stutter-free speech.

The clinician and Ms. L discussed the week ahead, and Ms. L agreed to continue structured and unstructured treatment. The clinician asked Ms. L to monitor fluctuations in Dean's SRs across each day, particularly noting his highest SR.

Clinic Visit 9

▶ **Within-Clinic Speech Measure: 3%SS**

Dean's preschool teacher commented to Ms. L that Dean seemed more confident when talking in a group situation. Ms. L reported that her SRs reflected Dean's typical speech each day, although he also had short periods each day in which SRs were 1 or 2. Structured treatment was done on 5 days, and unstructured treatment occurred each day. Ms. L reported that she praised his stutter-free speech twice as often as she asked him to self-correct stutters.

The clinician recommended that Ms. L do structured treatment when Dean's SR was 4 or higher in the week ahead, and unstructured treatment when his SR was 3 or lower.

Clinic Visit 10

▶ **Within-Clinic Speech Measure: 2%SS**

Ms. L reported that Dean's stutters were all syllable repetitions. Dean requested to do a "talking game" on two occasions, so they had done structured treatment on those days. Unstructured treatment occurred each day, and Ms. L said that she had used contingencies for stutter-free speech four or fives times more often than contingencies for stutters. Dean spontaneously self-corrected stutters each day, and commented to his mother about his smooth talking. Ms. L consistently praised each self-correction, and agreed with Dean's spontaneous self-evaluations of stutter-free speech.

The clinician asked Ms. L to listen to two 10-minute samples of Dean's speech in conversations during the week ahead, and count the number of stutters in them.

Clinic Visit 11

▶ **Within-Clinic Speech Measure: 2%SS**

Ms. L reported that Dean was sometimes stutter-free for up to 1 hour in conversations with her or with his preschool teacher. In the two tape recorded conversation samples, she had counted three stutters in the first sample, and one stutter in the second. All stutters were syllable repetitions.

The clinician and Ms. L discussed treatment for the week ahead. They agreed that Ms. L would continue treatment in unstructured conversations and would conduct structured treatment only if Dean asked for it.

Clinic Visit 12

▶ **Within-Clinic Speech Measure: 1%SS**

Ms. L reported that Dean was stutter-free for at least part of each day, as well as for 2 entire days. Ms. L used verbal contingencies for stutter-free speech many times each day, and prompted Dean to self-correct some stutters. She reported that he spontaneously self-corrected his other stutters.

The clinician described Stage 2 to Ms. L and explained that Dean would probably progress to it in a few weeks. In the meantime, she should continue treatment in unstructured conversations.

Clinic Visit 13

▶ **Within-Clinic Speech Measure: 0%SS**

Ms. L reported that Dean's speech was mostly stutter-free. She said that she did not always remember to acknowledge and praise stutter-free speech as often as in previous weeks, but that Dean would self-evaluate his stutter-free speech once or twice on most days. The clinician suggested that Dean's next clinic visit appointment be in 2 weeks, and that he would progress to Stage 2 if his SR remained stable.

Clinic Visit 14

▶ Within-Clinic Speech Measure: 0%SS

Ms. L confirmed that Dean rarely stuttered during the past 2 weeks. She listened to two 10-minute samples of his speech each week, and heard no more than one stutter in each of them. The clinician confirmed that Dean was ready to progress to Stage 2, and discussed with Ms. L the speech criteria and schedule of his future clinic visits. The clinician recommended that Ms. L continue treatment without changes until Dean's first Stage 2 clinic visit.

Stage 2

The standard program criteria and schedule were used (see Chapter 7). The second visit was repeated because Dean's speech was measured at 2%SS during the conversation in clinic, and consequently did not meet program criteria. Other than that, Dean met all Stage 2 requirements, and was discharged 46 weeks after starting Stage 2.

Chapter 10

Special Case Studies

Sally Hewat, Vanessa Harris, and Elisabeth Harrison

Most children attending our clinics for stuttering treatment progress through the Lidcombe Program in a straightforward manner. However, some children have additional problems or unusual circumstances that affect their progress. The challenge for their clinicians is to adjust treatment for their particular circumstances while maintaining the integrity of the Lidcombe Program. In this chapter we identify challenges related to specific client groups and investigate their impact on treatment delivery and progress.

Children have unique personal characteristics and family circumstances. We routinely consider these so that we can deliver the Lidcombe Program in the most effective and efficient manner. Delivering the Lidcombe Program to clients with difficult circumstances involves similar considerations. Potential challenging variables may be identified during the initial assessment session, and subsequent treatment can be planned accordingly. Other challenging variables may become evident only after treatment commences or even much later in the treatment process. Whenever the challenges are identified, it is the clinician's role to assess the effect of these variables on treatment progress and outcome. This is done most simply by considering the effect such variables may have on the various components of the Lidcombe Program. Some examples follow.

Training parents to deliver treatment will be different for parents of children from a non–English speaking background, and for parents of children with multiple problems. Parent training is also affected by irregular clinic attendance that may result from illness of a family member, busy parent schedules, unusual parent learning styles, and the presence of distracting siblings during clinic visits.

Measurement may be affected by limited contact between the parent and child, which can occur for many reasons. Two common reasons are a child's full-day attendance at day care and being part of a busy or large family. The measurement process also needs to be carefully considered when children speak more than one language, especially if they speak only one language with their parent and consequently their stuttering severity in the other language may not be measured. Using speech measures to track changes in stuttering severity is especially important for children with concomitant medical, speech, and language problems. Changes in stuttering severity may be directly related to the concomitant problems.

Treatment involves parents delivering verbal contingencies during structured and unstructured conversations. Delivering verbal contingencies to a very shy or sensitive child is very different than delivering contingencies to a talkative or extroverted child. Delivery of structured treatment is easily affected by the parent–child relationship, which can be under stress for many reasons, including a history of unsuccessful speech therapy, busy families, or child behavior problems, to name a few. Determining appropriate treatment for a child with concomitant speech or language problems also raises unique and challenging issues.

During Stage 2, the challenging case will require particular consideration. Children with a concomitant speech or language disorder may require slower withdrawal of stuttering treatment while treatment for their other speech or language disorders is introduced. Children from busy families, particularly those children with a history of inconsistent Stage 1 treatment, may also need closer monitoring and more systematic withdrawal of treatment during Stage 2.

Many circumstances have the potential to affect the routine delivery of the Lidcombe Program. Through the case examples discussed in this chapter, we demonstrate that treatment can be just as effective if challenges are identified and strategies developed in response to them. If unusual circumstances are not accounted for, unrealistic expectations may be set by the clinician and conveyed to the parent. With each child in treatment with the Lidcombe Program, the clinician looks for progress, even though it may be slower in children with special circumstances. As long as progress occurs, the clinician has a good indication that treatment is being delivered effectively. For many of the special cases we describe, it would be reasonable to expect treatment to take longer than usual. However, as demonstrated in some of the following case studies, more time is not always necessary.

We have identified particular client groups that present with typical stuttering and case histories, along with additional issues that complicate their stuttering treatment. For example, children who stutter may also have speech or language problems, medical problems, behavior problems, sensitivity, shyness, or talkativeness; have developmental delays; come from non–English speaking families; or attend full-time child care or educational settings. Each of these child–parent conditions can potentially affect delivery of each Lidcombe Program component. In the rest of this chapter, we consider each client group and the effect of these complicating issues. The case studies illustrate how the clinician identified the issues, solved problems with the parents, and adapted components of the Lidcombe Program to achieved satisfactory treatment outcomes with the Lidcombe Program. The names of the children have been changed.

Children with Other Speech and Language Problems

A number of children who come to the clinic for stuttering have other speech or language problems. These problems may include phonological and articulation disorders, language delays or disorders, voice disorders, or dyspraxia.

The effect of concomitant speech and language problems on delivery of the Lidcombe Program varies from child to child, depending on the circumstances of each child and family. Timing of intervention, setting priorities for treatment, the effect of previous treatment, the child's response to previous treatment, and the involvement and motivation of parents are all issues to be considered. Deciding to intervene for stuttering first among many disorders may be considered, although this is not always the most appropriate decision. Many variables need to be considered, including severity and impact of all the presenting problems on the child's communication, short- and long-term prognosis with and without intervention, the effect of treating one disorder on the other disorder(s), the child's reaction to the problems, and the parents' concerns.

In the following two case studies, we describe the implementation of the Lidcombe Program for two children, in the first case before and in the other case concurrent with intervention for speech and language problems.

Jacob

Background and Assessment

Jacob was age 4 years 1 month when he first came to the clinic. He was the second youngest of five children and lived with his mother and stepfather on weekdays, and with his father on weekends. Jacob's preschool teacher referred him for speech pathology assessment, as she was concerned about his speech and language development. Assessment results showed him to have severe stuttering, moderate phonological disorder, and delayed language development. The clinician recommended that Jacob begin stuttering treatment first as this was his most severe communication problem.

Two challenging issues were identified during the initial consultation and were discussed with Jacob's mother before commencing the Lidcombe Program. First, the possible effect between his speech and language problems and stuttering treatment progress required consideration. The clinician thought that although Jacob's stuttering severity might increase as he used longer and more complex language, it was also possible that his speech and language skills might improve during treatment with the Lidcombe Program. Second, the level of involvement in treatment by Jacob's separated mother and father would need to be considered. It was mutually agreed that Jacob's mother, Ms. B, would attend weekly clinic visits, collect speech measures, and conduct treatment during the week. His father would collect severity ratings (SRs) during Jacob's weekend visits, and the situation would be reviewed regularly.

Stage 1

Treatment commenced the following week. Ms. B and Jacob's father attended the first two clinic visits. This was arranged to ensure that the SRs collected at home by both parents were reliable and valid. During the second clinic visit, Ms. B learned to conduct structured treatment. Initially, the clinician demonstrated treatment using picture books as stimuli. This simple activity was chosen so that Jacob could produce more stutter-free utterances, while enabling the clinician and his mother to understand what he said. This activity was also well within Jacob's language abilities. Praise for stutter-free speech was initially introduced, along with tangible rewards to provide more structure for the activity and to indicate to Jacob the beginning and end of the activity. During the first few weeks, Ms. B was instructed to use contingencies for stutter-free speech only. The clinician felt that it was important to ensure that the parental contingencies were specifically for stutter-free speech. No contingencies were used for Jacob's speech sounds and language.

Contingencies for stuttered speech were introduced during the fifth clinic visit, and SRs increased from 3 to 5 during the following week. The clinician observed Ms. B conducting structured treatment and noticed many requests for clarification even on stutter-free utterances. Ms. B said that she did this to increase the clarity of Jacob's speech, even though she could understand him. The clinician reiterated that verbal contingencies were to be for stutter-free or stuttered speech only for the time being, and that treatment to increase Jacob's intelligibility would begin in the future if necessary.

Jacob's SRs decreased over the following weeks, and praise for stutter-free speech was introduced in unstructured conversations. When SRs were consistently 3, correction in unstructured situations was also introduced. His SRs continued to decrease, and Jacob reached Stage 2 speech criteria 17 weeks after starting Stage 1.

Stage 2

Initially in Stage 2, Jacob's parents reported hearing occasional stutters, especially when he was very excited or tired. Therefore, one unusual feature of Jacob's Stage 2 schedule was to have four biweekly clinic visits before moving on to monthly visits. Jacob's records show that although he continued to meet criteria, he also continued to stutter occasionally through the first 5 months of Stage 2. Unstructured treatment was systematically and slowly withdrawn over 3 months. When Jacob was discharged 14 months after starting Stage 2, his parents confirmed that they had heard no stuttering at all for 6 months.

Toward the end of Stage 2, Jacob attended a formal speech and language assessment at another clinic. Results indicated that his language was within normal limits, and he had a mild phonological disorder. He commenced treatment for this 2 weeks before his final Stage 2 clinic visit. Ms. B phoned our clinic several months later and reported that Jacob had successfully finished treatment, was enjoying "big school," and remained stutter-free.

Linda

Background and Assessment

Linda was age 4 years 6 months when she came to the clinic with her mother, Ms. M, for assessment. Ms. M reported that Linda had been stuttering for the past 12 months, and during the last 2 months it had become more severe. Linda's stuttering consisted of fixed postures of long duration with rising pitch and volume, and she frequently gave up talking altogether when she could not get out what she wanted to say. On one sample of her speech, she had a rating of 19% syllables stuttered (19%SS). The clinician found much of Linda's speech unintelligible, although Ms. M understood most of what Linda said.

The clinician attempted to administer a speech and language screening assessment but could not complete this due to the severity of Linda's stuttering. Ms. M and the clinician discussed treatment priorities and agreed to start the Lidcombe Program and to monitor Linda's speech and language.

Stage 1

Linda started Stage 1 three weeks later and her initial SRs were 8 and 9. Structured treatment was introduced using simple pictures and games. Linda's speech was consistently intelligible in short utterances when she was also consistently stutter-free. After 3 weeks of treatment, Ms. M commented that Linda no longer reacted to her stuttering with frustration, and most of her stutters were short fixed postures with audible airflow and syllable repetitions. Over the following weeks, Linda started using longer stutter-free utterances in treatment, and her speech became more intelligible to the clinician. Unstructured treatment was introduced during Linda's fifth clinic visit, and structured treatment was withdrawn over the next 3 weeks. Linda continued to make progress, and met Stage 1 speech criteria at her 12th clinic visit.

Stage 2

Linda's Stage 2 schedule started with three biweekly clinic visits, followed by a typical Stage 2 schedule that continued for 9 months. Ms. M continued to praise Linda's stutter-free speech once or twice per day during the first month of Stage 2.

Five months after Linda started Stage 2, she began speech and language therapy at a clinic near her preschool. At a subsequent Stage 2 clinic visit, Ms. M reported that there had been several 2- and 3-day periods when Linda's stuttering severity had increased to an SR of 3. On each occasion, Ms. M reintroduced unstructured therapy, and severity returned to an SR of 1 within 2 days. Ms. M felt that these increases in SR occurred with developments in Linda's speech and language. Linda met all speech criteria at each subsequent clinic visit, and was discharged 11 months after starting Stage 2.

Summary: Children with Other Speech and Language Problems

In our experience, when children present to the clinic with stuttering and concommitant speech problems, language problems, or both, the decision about which problem to treat first needs to be made carefully. Given the time-consuming nature of parent training in the Lidcombe Program, it is not viable to treat stuttering at the same time as other speech and language problems. Another important issue is that parents need to be clear about the nature of the treatment and treatment goals, and to understand the speech disorder being treated. It would cause problems if, for example, parents confused stuttering with incorrect productions of speech sounds, or considered both problems when assigning SRs to their child's speech. We typically implement the Lidcombe Program first, and monitor the child's speech and language. Treatment for other problems can then commence, or recommence, during Stage 2.

Once a decision has been made to implement the Lidcombe Program, it is important to consider the relative strengths and weaknesses of the child's speech or language abilities when structuring stuttering treatment activities. These activities need to change as the child's speech and language develops. It is particularly important to ensure with these children that parental verbal contingencies are specific, and that there is no confusion for the children about what is being acknowledged or praised or what they are being asked to self-correct.

Children with Medical Problems

In our experience, the Lidcombe Program may be used successfully with children who have serious medical problems. Children treated in our clinics include those with asthma, diabetes, attention-deficit (with or without hyperactivity) disorder (ADD or ADHD), depression, and chronic infections (e.g., otitis media, tonsillitis).

The impact of these illnesses on stuttering treatment will vary according to the complexity of the medical problems, and children's and families' responses to them. Among the most common problems for sick children are lethargy and lack of sleep. These result in parents and children having few opportunities for stuttering treatment. Another frequent issue is children missing many stuttering clinic visits due to medical appointments with local doctors, specialist physicians, and other health professionals. This results in parents having limited opportunities for consultation with clinicians about solving treatment problems. There are also more complex interactions of illness and stuttering treatment. Examples of these are stuttering severity that increases with recurrent illness or with doses of essential medications. The following case studies describe stuttering treatment for two children whose medical problems affected implementation of the Lidcombe Program.

Juan

Background and Assessment

Juan was age 4 years 3 months and the youngest of four children. At assessment Juan's mother, Ms. K, described his stuttering as cyclical, and estimated that he had been stuttering for 18 months. She reported that Juan had recently developed severe asthma, and had been admitted to the hospital during the most recent episode. However, Juan was well at the time of his assessment. Stuttering rate in the clinic was 5%SS, and his mother gave this particular speech sample an SR of 4. She said that severity would frequently be 6, or even 7, when Juan was playing with his younger brother.

Stage 1

At the first clinic visit, the clinician asked Ms. K to keep a daily record of Juan's SRs and days when he had asthma. This allowed Ms. K and the clinician to identify possible links between Juan's stuttering severity and his asthma. The clinician also introduced structured treatment, and Ms. K agreed to do daily treatment.

Juan was unable to attend three of his next four clinic visits, as he was unwell with asthma. His SRs tended to be 1 or 2 points higher than usual on days when he had asthma. Ms. K said that she was reluctant to do treatment with Juan on the days when he was unwell, as she was very worried about his health. The clinician suggested keeping treatment in structured conversation simple, where Ms. K could look at simple picture books with Juan and acknowledge and praise stutter-free speech as it occurred.

Juan was unable to attend the next two clinic visits, again due to illness. Although Ms. K was keen for Juan to continue stuttering treatment, she said that her greatest concern was managing his asthma and getting it stabilized. The clinician suggested recommencing treatment at a later date when Juan's health improved, and Ms. K agreed.

Five months later Ms. K contacted the clinician again, and Juan started stuttering treatment for the second time. Ms. K recorded Juan's SR and asthma each day, and found that his SRs were still higher on days when he was unwell. However, his asthma was under better control due to a new medication. Ms. K therefore was able to do treatment on most days and Juan subsequently progressed through Stage 1 without difficulty. There were 4 days on which he was too unwell to do treatment. Juan achieved speech criteria for entering Stage 2 after 17 clinic visits.

Stage 2

Juan's Stage 2 schedule was for a 16-month period, during which he attended the clinic at intervals of 2, 2, 4, 4, 4, 6, 6, and 8 weeks. The clinician and Ms. K contacted each other by phone after a further 8 and 16 weeks. During the first 7 months of Stage 2, Ms. K described Juan's speech as "less fluent" during episodes of asthma, although she did not think he stuttered. When his asthma was controlled, his speech "sounded better." Ms. K audiotaped samples of Juan's speech when he was "less fluent," and the clinician agreed that he was not stuttering, although he spoke more slowly and with more frequent pauses than was typical for him. Juan was discharged following the final phone conversation.

Brent

Background and Assessment

Brent was assessed 6 months after the onset of his stuttering, when his age was 3 years 6 months. Two months prior to assessment, there was a marked increase in his stuttering severity, and Brent started to talk louder than normal when he stuttered. There was a strong family history of stuttering: His mother and maternal grandfather both stuttered. During the assessment, a sample of Brent's speech was measured as 7%SS. His mother, Ms. C, also reported that Brent had been recently diagnosed with diabetes. Brent began the Lidcombe Program 3 weeks later.

Stage 1

At the first clinic visit, Ms. C reported that Brent was having twice daily insulin injections, as well as finger-prick blood tests six times per day. Brent was unable to attend his next clinic visit due to a medical appointment, so Ms. C agreed to collect daily SRs over 2 weeks. Brent's next two clinic visits were straightforward, and Ms. C learned how to use verbal contingencies in structured and unstructured conversations. Brent was unable to attend again for the following 2 weeks due to medical appointments.

At Brent's next clinic visit, Ms. C reported that his SRs had generally decreased. She also commented that his moods changed when his blood sugar levels were unstable and this seemed to correlate with increased SRs. Subsequently, Brent's doctor increased his insulin dosage, which had the effect of stabilizing his blood sugar level. Two days later there was a marked decrease in Brent's SRs.

Ms. C reported that although Brent's moods were still affected by blood sugar fluctuations, she was usually able to make treatment an enjoyable activity for Brent each day. However, around 10 weeks after starting Stage 1, Brent became annoyed with his six daily blood sugar tests. Ms. C reported that he had begun to upset her by wiping blood on both of them each time he had finger-prick tests. Although she was distressed by this behavior and anxious about Brent's reaction to the blood tests, she also found that Brent enjoyed his stuttering treatment and so she continued it each day. She avoided using verbal contingencies for stutter-free or stuttered speech during conversations with Brent about his behavior during finger-prick tests.

Ms. C reported that, rather than hindering her delivery of speech treatment, the diabetes management routine helped her understand how to adjust the level of treatment. That is, she used the SRs to decide on what "dosage" of treatment was needed, just as she needed to take blood sugar readings to determine the appropriate level of insulin that Brent required. Brent continued to progress through the program, and 19 weeks after he started Stage 1, he met the speech criteria for entry into Stage 2.

Stage 2

Brent progressed through Stage 2, meeting speech criteria at all clinic visits. Ms. C reported that she had gradually decreased contingencies for stutter-free speech over the first 2 months of Stage 2. No verbal contingencies were necessary for stuttered speech, as SRs were consistently 1. Brent was discharged 8 months after starting Stage 2.

Summary: Children with Medical Problems

Our experience is that children who have medical problems progress through Stage 1 more slowly than usual. Clinic visits may be attended less regularly, and parents may not have as many opportunities to conduct daily treatment due to children being unwell, needing to attend medical appointments, or receiving medical treatments. Creative problem solving with parents can assist them to overcome barriers to consistent treatment. Parents may also benefit from the clinician's support and encouragement to maintain treatment in difficult circumstances.

Realistic expectations are necessary when negotiating the timing of treatment with parents of children who have chronic or significant medical problems. It may be best to delay stuttering treatment until the child's illness is managed at a level where it will not negatively affect treatment. Continuing to attempt treatment in circumstances where it is not effective can be frustrating for the clinician, parents, and children. In addition, parents and children are likely to find treatment difficult to sustain if it has been pursued unsuccessfully for a long time. Sometimes, delaying treatment for a short time produces a better long-term outcome.

Children from Non–English Speaking Backgrounds

In our experience, Lidcombe Program treatment for children from non–English speaking backgrounds may not differ substantially from that for English-speaking children. Cultural and linguistic issues arise in treatment of many clients, regardless of whether they speak English or another language.

Maria

Background and Assessment

When Maria first came to our clinic for an initial assessment, she was 4 years 2 months of age and had been stuttering for 13 months. Her mother reported that Maria spoke Portuguese, whereas her parents and older brother (age 7 years) spoke Portuguese and English. All family members spoke Portuguese at home. Maria recently had started attending a local English-speaking preschool, and they noticed she already was using English words and phrases in her spontaneous speech.

Although the assessment session was conducted in English, the clinician was able to identify Maria's stutters while she talked with her mother in Portuguese. Her stuttering consisted of both repeated movements and fixed postures with audible airflow. Maria's mother, Ms. N, rated Maria's stuttering as SR 5, and reported that this was typical of her speech during the previous 3 weeks.

Stage 1

The clinician explained to Ms. N how to make severity ratings and how to do the treatment, and then role-played structured treatment with her. They discussed verbal contingencies for stutter-free and stuttered speech and identified Portuguese terms that Ms. N could use. Ms. N then did structured treatment with Maria, speaking in Portuguese. The clinician was able to recognize Ms. N's words used for verbal contingencies and therefore confirm that verbal contingencies were being used correctly. Maria seemed to enjoy the treatment and would look at the clinician and smile when her mother praised her stutter-free speech.

Maria's treatment was conducted at home in Portuguese, and the clinician and Ms. N talked in English at the clinic visits. Maria progressed through Stage 1 without difficulty, and her SRs showed a steady improvement from week to week. She met criteria for entering Stage 2 after nine clinic visits.

Stage 2

At Maria's fourth clinic visit, 12 weeks after starting Stage 2, Ms. N reported that Maria had started to stutter when speaking English at preschool and with friends. Her English language skills had developed quickly and she was able to talk in connected sentences, using Portuguese words when she was unsure of English vocabulary. Ms. N reported SRs of 1 when Maria was speaking Portuguese and of 3 to 4 when she was speaking English. The clinician and Ms. N agreed that Maria would return to Stage 1.

Stage 1

The clinician recommended that Ms. N collect two daily SRs, one for Maria's speech in Portuguese, and the second for English. She also recommended that Ms. N continue giving Maria verbal contingencies for stutter-free speech during conversations in Portuguese and do structured treatment in English. Ms. N was a little reluctant at first to do treatment in English at home as the family spoke only Portuguese there. The clinician suggested that Ms. N and Maria could have a "special time," perhaps 15 to 20 minutes each day, when they would speak English while doing structured treatment. The clinician suggested that they would speak Portuguese during the rest of the day, and that treatment would occur in natural conversations. Ms. N agreed to do this, and treatment was conducted accordingly each day. Two weeks later, SRs had reduced to 1 and 2 when Maria was speaking English and remained at 1 when speaking Portuguese. Ms. N introduced treatment in unstructured conversations, in English, for a 20-minute period per day, and Maria's SRs reduced again to become consistently 1 over several weeks. Maria entered Stage 2 again after seven clinic visits.

Stage 2

A Stage 2 schedule was devised for Maria that took into account her treatment history and the fact that she was still learning English. While standard speech criteria were used, her schedule of clinic visits continued for 14 months. Ms. N brought separate 10-minute audiotape recordings of Maria speaking in Portuguese and in English to each clinic visit. Ms. N reported occasional minor relapses early in Stage 2, and she managed these successfully between clinic visits. Maria successfully achieved speech criteria at each clinic visit, and was discharged after her 10th Stage 2 clinic visit.

Ahmad

Background and Assessment

Ahmad was age 4 years 1 month when he attended the clinic with his mother, Ms. B, for stuttering assessment. He was the second youngest of 13 children, 10 of whom lived at home with their parents. Two of Ahmad's older brothers had successfully completed courses of speech therapy for stuttering.

Ahmad spoke Arabic with his parents and English with his brothers and sisters and at school. He said that he preferred speaking English, and that English was probably his stronger language. His parents understood only a few English words. Consequently, an Arabic interpreter attended the assessment and all subsequent clinic visits to assist their communication with the clinician.

Ahmad's stuttering was severe and consisted of repeated movements and fixed postures with audible airflow, often accompanied by audible inhalations. The clinician and Ms. B were able to identify Ahmad's stutters in both Arabic and English. The clinician could not measure %SS when Ahmad spoke Arabic, as it was difficult to identify syllable boundaries. SRs were used to measure samples of Ahmad's speech in the clinic, in both languages. Ms. B and the clinician agreed that his SR was 7 in English and 9 in Arabic. Ms. B reported that these samples were typical, and that Ahmad usually stuttered more severely when speaking Arabic.

Stage 1

The clinician contacted the interpreter service several weeks before Ahmad's first Stage 1 clinic visit. The purpose of this was to book several consecutive weekly appointments with the same interpreter at a time that was convenient for Ms. B to attend with Ahmad while her older children were in school. There were several advantages in having the same interpreter attend the first Stage 1 clinic visits. First, Ms. B and the interpreter were able to establish rapport. Second, as the interpreter became more familiar with stuttering, speech measures, and treatment, he was able to give helpful, detailed information to the clinician about Ahmad's Arabic speech and language.

At the first appointment, the clinician, Ms. B, and the interpreter discussed and agreed on terminology that was meaningful to Ms. B and Ahmad. It was agreed that stutters would be called "bumps," and that Ms. B would praise Ahmad's stutter-free speech by saying "Bravo!"

The clinician then demonstrated structured treatment with Ahmad, in English, and the interpreter sat beside Ms. B and interpreted for her. Ahmad was distracted by hearing two simultaneous conversations, and continually looked at the interpreter, then his mother, then the clinician, unsure of whom to talk to or which language to use. Ms. B said she understood generally what to do, so the clinician suggested that she continue treatment with Ahmad, speaking Arabic. The clinician and interpreter took care to sit out of Ahmad's direct sight in order to minimize distraction. Ms. B used verbal contingencies for stutter-free speech, and Ahmad produced consistently stutter-free phrases while they talked together about a book. Ahmad enjoyed the activity a great deal, and said several times that he wanted to "do it more."

Over the following weeks, Ahmad made slow progress. He continued daily treatment sessions with his mother and continued to enjoy these greatly. As severity decreased to SRs of 3 (English) and 4 (Arabic) and treatment became less structured, Ms. B found it difficult to give verbal contingencies in natural conversations. There were several reasons for this. First, Ms. B was the mainstay of an extremely busy household; second, Ahmad frequently spoke English at home and Ms. B had to monitor his speech more carefully to hear stutters; and third, Ahmad spent a lot of time at home playing with his siblings rather than talking with his mother.

The clinician discussed with Ms. B the possibility that one of Ahmad's older siblings conduct treatment with him. Ms. B suggested Ahmad's 15-year-old sister, Rania, because they got on well and Rania liked to help look after her younger brothers and sisters. Ahmad's weekly appointment time was changed so that Rania could attend clinic visits with Ahmad and Ms. B.

The clinician and Ms. B demonstrated treatment in natural conversations, in Arabic and English, and Rania immediately showed a good understanding of what she was to do. Ahmad was delighted to have his big sister helping him with "bumps" and acknowledging and praising his stutter-free speech. Ms. B agreed that she would also continue to praise Ahmad's stutter-free Arabic speech in unstructured conversations with her. She also suggested that Rania could earn extra weekly allowance for helping Ahmad. This treatment routine was effective and Ahmad's SR dropped in both languages.

Several weeks later, when his SRs were 2 to 3, Rania reported that some of Ahmad's other siblings had started asking him to self-correct his stuttered speech. Ms. B had not been aware of this as the children did this during play, when they spoke English. Ahmad was annoyed by his sibling's comments, so the clinician requested that they be asked to stop their comments, which they did. Ahmad achieved speech criteria for entering Stage 2 after 24 clinic visits.

Stage 2

Four months after Ahmad started Stage 2, Ms. B went to Lebanon for 2 months and neither his father nor adult siblings could bring him to clinic visits. The clinician and Ms. B discussed alternatives to clinic visits, and agreed that the clinician would phone Rania every 4 weeks, check Ahmad's progress, and monitor severity. Ms. B agreed to contact the clinician and continue Stage 2 when she returned. Ahmad met speech criteria for each clinic visit, although Rania reported that his SRs were occasionally 2 or 3 while his mother was away. Ahmad finished Stage 2 after 12 months.

Summary: Children from Non–English Speaking Backgrounds

The parent training component of the Lidcombe Program involves, among other things, verbal explanations and detailed communication between the clinician and parent throughout Stages 1 and 2. In cases where parents require an interpreter at each clinic visit, we expect Stage 1 to take longer than usual because everything needs to be said twice. However, even parents with functional English skills may require assistance from interpreters at some clinic visits. We have found that misunderstanding of a minor piece of information can lead to confusion that extends the duration of treatment.

Cultural differences will influence how parents interact with their children, and consequently the way parents deliver treatment. For example, in some cultures it is not considered appropriate to praise children. Instead, correct behavior is expected of children, and so rewards and praise are redundant. However, rather than seeing cultural differences as barriers to successful treatment, we find them an enjoyable challenge because we work in communities that are culturally and linguistically diverse. In our day-to-day clinical practice, we work with individual parents to determine culturally appropriate ways to acknowledge and praise their children's stutter-free speech and deliver verbal contingencies for their stuttered speech.

For stuttering children who speak two languages, our experience is that treatment delivered in one language will often result in reduced stuttering in the second language. However, it may be necessary for parents to deliver treatment in both languages. If there is a slower response to treatment in one language, it is often due to the amount of treatment delivered in that language. For example, the parent may be unable to deliver sufficient treatment, as either child or parent favors one language over the other. In Ahmad's case, his mother was able to identify his stutters in English, but she spent limited time with him while he spoke English. Therefore, verbal contingencies were delivered inconsistently, and possibly incorrectly, in English. Collecting SRs for each language provides an effective way to monitor any differences in stuttering across time.

Sensitive or Shy Children

Presenting verbal contingencies can be problematic for parents whose children are shy or sensitive about being the focus of attention. A sensitive child may react adversely to contingencies for stuttered or stutter-free speech. These children may also interact differently with clinicians than with their parents. A shy child may not interact freely in a clinical situation at all. For these children, collecting valid speech measures and demonstrating treatment in the clinic are especially difficult.

The following case studies provide examples of issues with shy and sensitive children when implementing the Lidcombe Program. The case studies highlight how clinicians and parents worked together with these children to achieve successful treatment outcomes.

Samantha

Background and Assessment

Samantha, age 3 years 10 months, attended an assessment with her mother, Ms. T. Samantha lived at home with both parents and two older siblings. Samantha started stuttering 8 months previously, with what Ms. T described as repetitions, and her stuttering became progressively more severe until sometimes she was unable to say anything. Ms. T said Samantha had become increasingly frustrated by her speech. Samantha's father, his older sister, and Ms. T's brother all stuttered. Ms. T described Samantha as a "very quiet and shy child, especially around new people."

Ms. T brought an audiorecorded sample of Samantha's speech to the assessment, as she thought it unlikely that Samantha would speak with the clinician. The taped sample was measured as 7%SS, and her stutters were a combination of syllable repetitions and fixed postures with audible airflow. Ms. T rated the severity of this speech sample as an SR of 5, and said this was typical of Samantha's speech.

Stage 1

During the first clinic visit, the clinician explained to Ms. T how to measure severity and she agreed to collect daily SRs. The clinician attempted to build rapport with Samantha by playing with her and Ms. T, with toys that Samantha selected. Although Samantha seemed to enjoy this activity, she said very little.

Ms. T and Samantha attended the second clinic visit a week later. Samantha's average SR for the week was 6. The clinician was unable to obtain a valid sample of Samantha's speech in the clinic, as she said only a few single words. The clinician decided to obtain an alternative speech measure, and explained to Ms. T how to collect covert measures of stutters per minute of speaking time (SMST) at home. The clinician described for Ms. T how to do structured treatment, and demonstrated praise for stutter-free speech during play with Samantha. The clinician requested Ms. T to attempt a structured therapy activity at home each day with Samantha, and to stop if she showed any signs of not enjoying the activity. She also asked Ms. T to audiotape one structured treatment session.

A similar pattern of clinic visits continued for the next 5 weeks. Each week, Ms. T brought to the clinic visit (a) daily SRs, (b) an audiotaped sample of Samantha's speech or an SMST measure, and (c) an audiotaped sample of one or two structured therapy sessions. The clinician and Ms. T discussed the speech measures and treatment in detail, listened to the audiotapes, and discussed changes to treatment. Ms. T was able to do structured treatment with Samantha during clinic visits while the clinician observed through a one-way mirror and confirmed that treatment was appropriate and that Ms. T's verbal contingencies were accurate. Over these weeks, Samantha also started to talk more frequently with the clinician. Each week, Samantha brought something to show the clinician and would talk about it. Ms. T said that Samantha loved planning what to show the clinician, and they had long conversations about it on the day before each clinic visit. By the seventh clinic visit, Ms. T confirmed that Samantha's conversation was typical of her speech at home.

Although there was no dramatic change in Samantha's SR during the first 5 to 6 weeks of treatment, Ms. T reported that Samantha was using more stutter-free spontaneous speech during structured treatment. Ms. T introduced verbal contingencies for Samantha's stutter-free speech during unstructured conversations, and continued with daily structured treatment. During the eighth clinic visit, the clinician introduced contingencies for stuttered speech and recommended that Ms. T request Samantha to self-correct her stutters. Ms. T then praised the second utterance, which was stutter-free. The clinician recommended that Ms. T continue frequent contingencies for Samantha's stutter-free speech.

Samantha attended her next clinic visit 2 weeks later with Ms. T, her brother, and her sister. Ms. T reported a dramatic decrease in Samantha's stuttering, with SRs of 2 or 3 each day for the previous 2 weeks. Ms. T also reported that Samantha was stutter-free for longer periods of the day. During the clinic visit, while Samantha played and talked with her siblings, the clinician measured a long sample of her speech as 1.5%SS and SR 2. Ms. T confirmed that this was typical of her speech over the past week. The clinician recommended that Ms. T increase therapy in unstructured conversations with Samantha, and eliminate structured treatment altogether. After three more clinic visits, a total of 15 altogether, Samantha achieved requisite speech criteria to begin Stage 2.

Stage 2

Samantha attended all scheduled Stage 2 clinic visits, and achieved speech criteria at each one.

Bethany

Background and Assessment

Bethany attended our clinic for assessment when she was age 3 years 9 months, 18 months after onset of her stuttering. According to Bethany's mother, her stuttering began as repetitions and progressed to fixed postures. Ms. C reported that she used to stop Bethany when she stuttered and ask her to say the words slowly. However, Bethany had become frustrated with this so Ms. C stopped commenting on her stutters.

Bethany's stuttering was measured in the clinic as 9%SS. Ms. C gave Bethany's speech an SR of 6 and said that Bethany's most severe stuttering would be SR 10 and her least severe would be SR 3. Stuttering rate on an audiotape of Bethany's speech at home was 2.3%SS, and Ms. C gave this sample an SR of 3.

Stage 1

At the first clinic visit, Ms. C reported that Bethany's stutter had changed, and she now hesitated on the first words of some utterances "as if she didn't know what she wanted to say." Bethany still repeated and extended syllables as well, but overall she stuttered less frequently. Bethany would not speak while the clinician was in the room, and Ms. C said that Bethany was shy when meeting new people and when she was the focus of attention. The clinician explained various types of stutters to Ms. C—repetitions and fixed postures—and discussed with her how best to collect SRs in the following week. The clinician described treatment to Ms. C and they discussed how it could be conducted at home. They agreed to delay starting treatment until Bethany was more at ease in the clinic.

At the second and third clinic visits, it became evident that Bethany was avoiding speaking in the clinic, and she used a "baby voice" when she talked to the clinician. The clinician and Ms. C continued to play with Bethany and thereby help her to feel more comfortable in the clinic. During unstructured play, Ms. C twice attempted praise for stutter-free speech by saying, "That's sounding good," and on both occasions, Bethany started again to talk in her baby voice.

By her fifth clinic visit, Bethany talked naturally with the clinician. Ms. C was able to praise Bethany's stutter-free speech several times in a conversation about the toys Bethany brought with her to the clinic. A bingo game also worked well, and the clinician indirectly praised Bethany's stutter-free speech and continued with the conversation. Ms. C reported that treatment at home consisted of daily structured treatment while playing a game chosen each day by Bethany, and praise for Bethany's stutter-free speech was incorporated into unstructured conversations.

At the following clinic visit, Ms. C reported that Bethany's SRs were usually 3 or 4, and that her highest SR in the past week was 5. The clinician explained verbal contingencies for stuttered speech to Ms. C, and they discussed which contingencies to use with Bethany. Ms. C then did structured treatment with Bethany, and asked her to self-correct occasional stuttered words (e.g., "Can you say 'boat' again?"). Bethany consistently corrected the stuttered words, and Ms. C was able to do structured treatment with Bethany in an easy and relaxed manner. Ms. C agreed to request one self-correction during each structured activity at home and to use only praise during unstructured treatment.

During the following weeks, Bethany's SRs were still 3 to 5, but Ms. C reported hearing short periods of stutter-free speech on most days. Ms. C suggested that she could use more frequent contingencies for Bethany's stuttered speech as she felt that Bethany would respond to this now. Ms. C and Bethany played one of her favorite games, and Bethany conversed freely. Ms. C praised Bethany's stutter-free speech and asked her to self-correct each stutter, which Bethany did successfully and consistently. Over the following 4 weeks, Ms. C continued the same treatment and Bethany responded the same way. Her SRs decreased to 2 to 3. At a subsequent clinic visit, Ms. C reported that Bethany had started to spontaneously correct her stutters and then tell her mother that she had "fixed a bump."

Despite her obvious enjoyment of treatment with her mother, Bethany remained relatively shy and would talk freely with the clinician only at every second or third clinic visit. Ms. C confirmed that Bethany was naturally quiet and that her behavior during the clinic visits was completely natural.

During the final weeks of Stage 1, Ms. C made regular audiotapes of Bethany's speech at home. These recordings provided the clinician with several representative samples of Bethany's speech each week, and confirmed that Bethany had achieved speech criteria to begin Stage 2. Bethany did not speak consistently enough during clinic visits to be able to rely on speech measures from that situation. Bethany commenced Stage 2 after 23 clinic visits.

Stage 2

Audio- and videotaped speech samples were used throughout Stage 2 to determine Bethany's speech measures. Bethany achieved her Stage 2 speech criteria on each visit and completed Stage 2 in 10 months.

Summary: Sensitive or Shy Children

Because the Lidcombe Program is a parent-delivered treatment program, it is not essential to build a strong relationship between the child and clinician. The clinician's essential role is to train the parent, and it is the parent who needs to have a strong relationship with the child to conduct treatment successfully. If the clinician can obtain representative audio- or videotaped samples of the child's speech at home, and observe the parent and child conducting treatment, then the program can proceed without difficulty.

When treating quiet or shy children, we occasionally come across parents who need suggestions about how best to assist their child to feel comfortable talking. Parents may also need training to observe more subtle signs or changes in their child, which may indicate he or she is not comfortable with the interaction in some way. A shy child may withdraw from conversations if feeling under pressure to perform.

Other children are not necessarily shy, but are more accurately described as being sensitive to all verbal contingencies for their speech. In our experience, any negativity is most likely to be directed toward verbal contingencies for stuttered speech. However, we have treated a small number of children who have had a similar reaction to contingencies for stutter-free speech. This reaction occurred when praise was very frequent and too much attention was given to speech. It is worthwhile to remember that verbal contingencies can be simple acknowledgment of or a request for self-correction of stuttered speech, rather than praise.

Verbal contingencies for stuttered speech should be introduced with caution with all children, but particularly with children who are known to be sensitive or shy. We find that by initially limiting requests for self-correction to structured treatment, we can carefully watch each child's reaction and therefore reduce the likelihood of any negative effect.

Children of Working or Busy Parents

Involvement of the parent (or significant other) is essential to the success of treatment using the Lidcombe Program. Often at our clinic we treat children who (a) have two working or busy parents or (b) come from a split family and spend their time between two homes and sets of caregivers. Initial stages of treatment for these children are the most problematic. Finding sufficient time for effective parent training and consistent treatment in structured activities at home are often the biggest challenges for parents and clinician alike.

When working with these children and families, the clinician must be sure that parents understand what treatment entails and must clarify their willingness to commit time to treatment. The clinician also needs to understand the family's situation, assist parents realistically, and provide them with ideas about how to deliver effective treatment at home. Issues often involve frequency and consistency of parents' time with the child, pressured time when they are together, attending clinic visits consistently, collecting valid speech measures at home (difficult when the parent has limited contact with the child), and failure to complete Stage 2. The following case studies contain examples of clinicians negotiating with parents to deliver effective treatment.

Jamie

Background and Assessment

Jamie attended the clinic for stuttering assessment with his parents, Mr. and Ms. K, when he was age 3 years 11 months. Jamie's mother was a nurse and a shift worker; his father worked long hours as a computer programmer. Jamie was due to start preschool a few weeks after his assessment. Jamie had been stuttering for 10 months, and his parents said that severity had increased steadily since onset. A sample of Jamie's speech was measured as 8%SS and his parents rated the severity of this sample as 6. They reported that his stuttering severity usually fluctuated between SRs of 3 and 8.

Stage 1

Ms. K competently delivered daily treatment from the first clinic visit. During the first 6 weeks of treatment, Jamie responded well to treatment and his severity reduced from SRs of 7 and 8 to 4. During those weeks, his SRs increased slightly on two occasions. The first occasion was when his father went overseas for a week, and the second was when his mother started working night shifts. Jamie started preschool around the time of his seventh clinic visit, and after the eighth clinic visit his SRs were consistently 2. Ms. K was providing verbal contingencies for stutter-free and stuttered speech during unstructured conversations, and did structured treatment with Jamie if SRs were 3 or higher.

During the following week, Ms. K started a new job, which involved being on-call. The frequency of her work was unpredictable and she was usually notified the morning she had to work. Jamie spent these days being cared for by their neighbor. Then, Ms. K started working 4 and sometimes 5 days per week, and the frequency of treatment became intermittent. Jamie's SRs were consistently 1 to 2 points higher on days when Ms. K worked, and directly reflected therapy consistency.

Jamie's SRs remained at 4 for 5 consecutive weeks. The clinician and Ms. K discussed Jamie's treatment and came up with a few ideas designed to increase consistency of structured therapy. One suggestion was for Mr. and Ms. K to organize a time each day for Jamie to have structured treatment, with whichever parent was with him at that time. Another suggestion was for both parents to make daily SRs and to do unstructured treatment with Jamie. A third suggestion was to introduce a sticker chart. This served the dual purposes of reinforcing Jamie's stutter-free speech and being a visual reminder for Jamie's parents to do treatment with him. Jamie attended preschool only 1 day per week, so it was not an option to train his teacher to do treatment. Ms. K agreed that she needed to make Jamie's treatment a high priority, and she attempted during the following weeks to provide more consistent therapy.

Mr. K attended a few clinic visits with Jamie, as his workload had reduced. He also learned how to deliver verbal contingencies for stutter-free and stuttered speech during unstructured conversations. After 19 Stage 1 clinic visits, Jamie achieved speech criteria to move to Stage 2.

Stage 2

Ms. K was often unable to attend Stage 2 clinic visits. Consequently, the clinician agreed to replace some clinic visits with phone calls. Jamie met all speech criteria for 10 months of Stage 2. He was unable to attend his final clinic visit as his family moved overseas to live.

Veronica

Background and Assessment

Veronica attended the clinic with her parents, Mr. and Ms. W, for an assessment when she was age 3 years 7 months. Onset of her stuttering had occurred 18 months previously, and her parents reported that the severity of her stuttering had gradually increased since onset. At the assessment, Veronica's stuttering consisted of repeated movements and fixed postures with audible airflow. Stuttering rate was 12%SS, and SR was 7. Her parents estimated that this sample of speech was similar to her speech at home.

Stage 1

At the first clinic visit, the majority of Veronica's stutters were fixed postures with audible airflow, which were difficult for Ms. W and the clinician to identify unless they watched Veronica while she was talking. The clinician introduced SRs, and Ms. W agreed to chart severity daily. The clinician introduced treatment during a structured conversation, and Veronica was happy to participate. To achieve stutter-free speech, the clinician structured the conversation so that Veronica said phrases and occasional short sentences. Ms. W continued the conversation in the same manner. She agreed to do daily treatment during structured conversations with Veronica at home, to praise her stutter-free utterances, and not to use contingencies for stuttered speech.

In the following clinic session, Ms. W reported that she had done treatment only once, despite Veronica's asking to do it each day. Ms. W reported it had been an unusually busy time in her business, which she conducted from home. However, she did not think it would be a problem conducting daily therapy during the following week.

Veronica was unable to attend the following two appointments, and at the third clinic visit, Ms. W reported she and Veronica had conducted structured treatment only once in the past 3 weeks. Ms. W said that she had not previously realized how little time she actually spent with Veronica. The clinician and Ms. W discussed the family's daily routines and identified times each day when it would be possible to do treatment with Veronica. Ms. W decided that she could disengage her phone during treatment times so that they would not be interrupted. Ms. W was able to identify the components of treatment necessary to achieve stutter-free speech and she had a clear understanding of how treatment was meant to occur.

During the following weeks, Ms. W conducted treatment each day, and SRs decreased steadily to 2 and 3. Veronica's stuttering changed—she no longer had fixed postures, and most of her stutters were repeated movements. The clinician recommended that Ms. W adjust treatment so that most of it occurred during natural conversations. The clinician explained to Ms. W that it was likely that Veronica's SRs would increase again due to the cyclical nature of her stuttering. She also explained to Ms. W how to balance the amount of therapy conducted in structured and unstructured situations according to the SRs for any particular day.

Veronica was unable to attend the next scheduled clinic visit, as her mother was too busy at work.

At the next visit Ms. W reported severities of SR 1 and 2. Treatment during unstructured conversations had worked well in their busy routine, and Ms. W said that her major difficulty was remembering to be consistent throughout the day. She had thought about how she remembered to do things related to her business, and applied the same principle to remembering Veronica's treatment. She therefore put sticky yellow notes at strategic places around the house, where she could not fail to see them.

Veronica was unable to attend the clinic again the following week due to Ms. W's work commitments. At the next scheduled visit, Veronica's SRs remained at 1 and 2, and the clinician explained to Ms. W the requirements for Veronica to move on to Stage 2. Ms. W agreed to collect some videotaped speech samples over the following 2 weeks and to continue consistent treatment. Veronica met Stage 2 speech criteria 3 weeks later, which was after 17 Stage 1 clinic visits. She had been unable to attend 6 other appointments.

Stage 2

Veronica met all speech criteria for each of her scheduled Stage 2 clinic visits. Ms. W reported that occasionally SRs were 2 during the first 2 months of Stage 2, but she managed these herself between clinic visits. Veronica completed Stage 2 in 11 months.

Summary: Children of Working or Busy Parents

When using the Lidcombe Program with busy and working parents, it is important to assess each situation individually. Some parents, while working full time and running a household, are able to deliver effective therapy and fit treatment into already busy schedules. However, for other families treatment may be a lower priority and all aspects of treatment may need to be negotiated carefully. The negotiations may involve specific scheduling of structured treatment activities, and the setting of clear guidelines on the amount and consistency of treatment needed to reduce stuttering.

In some cases it is possible to train both parents—as well as caregivers, other relatives, or preschool teachers—to conduct treatment. The clinician needs to train each person, as this allows for clear lines of communication and ensures that the best possible treatment is presented to the child. It can be easier to involve others in treatment when it is delivered during unstructured conversations. However, the most important factor to consider when involving others in treatment is that the person is able to identify the child's stutter-free and stuttered speech accurately.

In cases where parents have a busy lifestyle, the clinician needs to facilitate parents' own problem solving, organizing, and scheduling so that the Lidcombe Program can be implemented. After all, if parents have not set the guidelines themselves, then they are unlikely to adhere to them. If there is a lack of progress or treatment is slower than expected, the clinician can communicate this to the parents and discuss the implications openly, being aware of the reasons for slow progress.

Conclusion

Children come to speech pathology clinics with unique personalities and situations, and their parents also have their own expectations, learning styles, and personal circumstances. In routine cases, these factors are taken into consideration throughout the collaborative relationship that develops between parent and clinician. In special cases, however, it is important for the clinician to consider and account for the effect of other problems on stuttering and on treatment. The clinician identifies challenging variables, and then assesses their impact on each treatment component. Strategies can then be applied to ensure that the Lidcombe Program is administered with integrity while ensuring the child's progress. We expect that, as with all other stuttering treatments, there will be children for whom, despite every effort, it is simply not possible for their parents to conduct treatment. These cases become obvious to both the parent and clinician during the course of treatment. A decision may be made to suspend or discontinue treatment until the family's situation changes and the parent is able to do treatment effectively. The parent training component is extremely important when solving problems in special cases. When parents understand the need for each treatment component, they may be more willing to make changes that are necessary to achieve therapy goals. If this is not possible, then they can make an informed decision to postpone treatment, cease treatment altogether, or seek another form of treatment.

Part IV

The Lidcombe Program Around the World

Chapter 11

Australia

Ann Packman, Isabelle Rousseau, Mark Onslow, Rebekah Dredge, Elisabeth Harrison, and Linda Wilson

There has been a strong tradition of behavioral treatments for stuttering in Australia. Until the last decade, however, this tradition has been associated almost exclusively with treatments for adolescents and adults. For example, the early research into the use of rhythmic speech and prolonged speech at the Prince Henry Hospital, Sydney, contributed greatly to the development and understanding of treatments based on these novel speech patterns (see Packman, Onslow, & Menzies, 2000). There were no documented behavioral treatments in Australia for preschool children prior to the publication of the first report, in 1990, of the operant treatment that was to become the Lidcombe Program (Onslow, Costa, & Rue, 1990). A number of subsequent publications have related to various aspects of the Lidcombe Program, particularly outcomes (see Chapter 1). The implementation of the program in this research has been standardized, and a manual for the program is available on the Web site of the Australian Stuttering Research Centre (www.fhs.usyd.edu.au/ASRC/).

Research into the Lidcombe Program in Australia, however, has been conducted mainly by the developers of the program, at the University of Sydney and the Stuttering Unit, Bankstown Health Service. This raises the issue of whether the program is used by Australian clinicians not directly associated with the Lidcombe/Bankstown team. This is an important issue, as it would seem a waste of resources to develop effective treatments unless they are accepted and implemented by the wider clinical community.

It should be noted at this point that the Lidcombe Program had humble origins (see Chapter 2). The program was not developed solely by academicians within a university, but rather as a collaboration between university researchers and clinicians who were working in a government-funded health center (see Chapter 2). Furthermore, the centers in which the program developed are in a low- to middle-class area of Sydney, with many ethnic minority groups. In other words, the development of the Lidcombe Program and the subsequent research into it have not occurred in an isolated or specialized environment. It seems likely, then, that 12 years after the initial report of Onslow et al. (1990), the Lidcombe Program has gained widespread acceptance among the clinical community in Australia.

There are a number of other reasons to think that the Lidcombe Program is more widely accepted and used around Australia. First, as discussed previously, there is a long tradition in Australia of behavioral approaches to the treatment of stuttering. For example, there is little evidence that the Australian clinical community was influenced to any great extent by Wendell Johnson's views on early stuttering (see Chapter 3). This position—that parents cause stuttering by mislabeling normal disfluencies as stuttering—had an enormous effect for more than 30 years on the treatment of the disorder in preschool children in other countries (for a discussion of cultural issues in early stuttering, see Attanasio, Onslow, & Menzies, 1996). It seems likely, then, that Australian clinicians face few theoretical or philosophical barriers to accepting the direct approach to stuttering embodied in the operant procedures of the Lidcombe Program.

Second, the Lidcombe Program is now taught widely in undergraduate university courses around the country. This suggests that many Australian clinicians would have been exposed to the program during their professional preparation.

Third, there is a vigorous program of continuing professional education in stuttering management in Australia. This program, which is conducted jointly by the Australian Stuttering Research Centre (ASRC) and the Stuttering Unit, incorporates workshops and teleconferences on the Lidcombe Program, and other treatments for stuttering, for practicing clinicians. This educational program is well patronized.

Finally, a consultative service available through the Stuttering Unit enables clinicians conducting the Lidcombe Program to consult with specialist clinicians about any difficulties they may be facing with implementing the program (see Chapter 8). This service is also well patronized by Australian clinicians.

All these reasons suggest that the Lidcombe Program is widely used in Australia. However, it is important to know how widespread that use is, whether clinicians in Australia consider the program to be effective, and whether it is the treatment of choice in Australia for preschool children who stutter. It is possible, for example, that the treatment procedures and format developed for the Lidcombe Program may not suit some speech pathology services in Australia. Many clinics in Australia have lengthy waiting lists for treatment, some clinics provide a consultative service only, and some deliver services predominantly via a parent-training model. Consequently, service delivery models in some areas may not accommodate the weekly treatment format of the program. For example, speech pathologists in the Sydney metropolitan area are moving away from the traditional service delivery model, which prescribes mainly in-clinic therapy delivery, toward providing services in a more natural environment, at least for children with language impairments (Cornick, 1996). Cornick showed that, at the time of that study, weekly contact with clients occurred for slightly less than half the caseloads of the speech pathologists surveyed.

One factor that affects the implementation of the Lidcombe Program in Australia is that vast tracts of the country are sparsely populated. At least 30% of Australian children live in remote areas where contact with speech pathologists is infrequent (Wilson, Lincoln, & Onslow, 2002; Wilson, Onslow, & Lincoln, 2002). These studies report that factors such as distance, transport disadvantage, socioeconomic factors, and limited accessibility of speech pathologists were perceived by clinicians to impair the quality of interventions for rural children. This was particularly the case for stuttering, where home programming and telephone contact were used to compensate for limited direct client contact.

During 1999, researchers at the ASRC conducted a survey of Australian speech pathologists to investigate their use of the Lidcombe Program (Rousseau, Packman, Onslow, & Robinson, 2000). The aim of the survey was to determine (a) the extent to which the program was used by Australian speech pathologists, (b) their level of satisfaction with the program, and (c) barriers to its implementation in Australian speech clinics. To this end, a questionnaire was sent to speech pathologists around Australia, asking a number of questions about their use of the program. A summary of the findings of this survey is presented in this chapter (the findings are presented in detail in Rousseau, Packman, Onslow, Dredge, & Harrison, 2002). This summary is followed by a brief overview of a program of research currently being conducted in Australia to develop a distance-intervention or telehealth model of delivery for the Lidcombe Program. The primary aim of this research is to improve the access to the Lidcombe Program of children and their families who live in remote and rural areas.

Survey of Australian Clinicians' Use of the Lidcombe Program

The Questionnaire

A questionnaire was mailed to 390 speech pathologists who were selected randomly by Speech Pathology Australia, the professional association of speech pathologists in Australia. Only members of the association who were registered as having children on their caseload were included. Questions had mostly multiple-choice answers; however, respondents were encouraged throughout the questionnaire to write comments. The questionnaire covered:

- Participants' workplace and caseloads
- Whether or not participants use the Lidcombe Program
- What participants use, if not the Lidcombe Program
- How participants use the Lidcombe Program
- How participants learned to use the Lidcombe Program
- Participants' ratings of the effectiveness of the Lidcombe Program
- General comments

Respondents

Twenty-two questionnaires were returned marked "address unknown." A further 277 clinicians sent back completed questionnaires, giving a response rate of 75%. This response rate is considered very satisfactory. Respondents were from all of the eight states and territories in Australia, approximately in proportion to their populations. Respondents were drawn from private practice, community health services, other community and disability service providers, and hospitals. The experience of the respondents with managing stuttering was not extensive, with almost half (49%) of the respondents having seen 1 to 10 cases in the previous 3 years. Respondents who used the Lidcombe Program reported that they had learned about it from a variety of sources—and typically from more than one source—including undergraduate professional preparation, conferences and workshops, journal articles, professional development in the workplace, observations, and the ASRC Web site. This information about respondents suggests that they were representative of the wider clinical community in Australia. They were primarily generalist clinicians, rather than specialists in treating stuttering, and had learned to do the Lidcombe Program in a variety of ways, although few had learned it directly from the developers of the program.

Use of the Lidcombe Program

Of the 277 respondents, 177 reported having treated stuttering in a preschool child in the previous 3 years. Of those, 154 (87%) reported that they routinely used the Lidcombe Program, or parts of it. When asked to rate the effectiveness of the program on a 5-point scale where 1 = *not effective* and 5 = *very effective*, most respondents marked 4 or 5 on the scale (see Figure 11.1). Of course, these ratings represent a subjective report of effectiveness and cannot be regarded as outcome measures.

Nonetheless, the findings suggest that the level of satisfaction of Australian clinicians with the Lidcombe Program is high.

Responses to other questions, however, indicated that only 55% of clinicians who used the Lidcombe Program actually used it in the way it is described in research publications or according to the treatment manual. In many cases, children and families did not attend the clinic each week, and Stage 2 was not implemented according to 68% of respondents who used the program.

These findings were somewhat unexpected. Although the findings suggest widespread use and acceptance of the program in Australia, less than half of those who use the program implement it in its entirety. The fact that many clinicians do not implement Stage 2 of the program is of concern. This part of the program is designed to maintain over time the low levels of stuttering severity achieved at the end of Stage 1 (see Chapter 7). This maintenance of beneficial treatment effects is particularly important for young children, given the variability over time of early stuttering, and the fact that stuttering can disappear completely in young children, only to reappear at some time—perhaps months—later. It is critical, then, to ensure that the low levels of stuttering observed at the completion of Stage 1 are in fact durable.

Of the 177 respondents who treated stuttering, 23 (13%) reported that they did not use the Lidcombe Program. Respondents were asked why they did not use it and were given a checklist of possibilities, including the option "other." The results, shown in Figure 11.2, indicate that a number of these respondents simply did not know how to use the Lidcombe Program. Respondents who did not use the Lidcombe Program were also asked what other treatments they used and were given a checklist with the option "other." The results are shown in Figure 11.3. The most commonly used treatment was environmental manipulation (see Chapter 3). Second most common

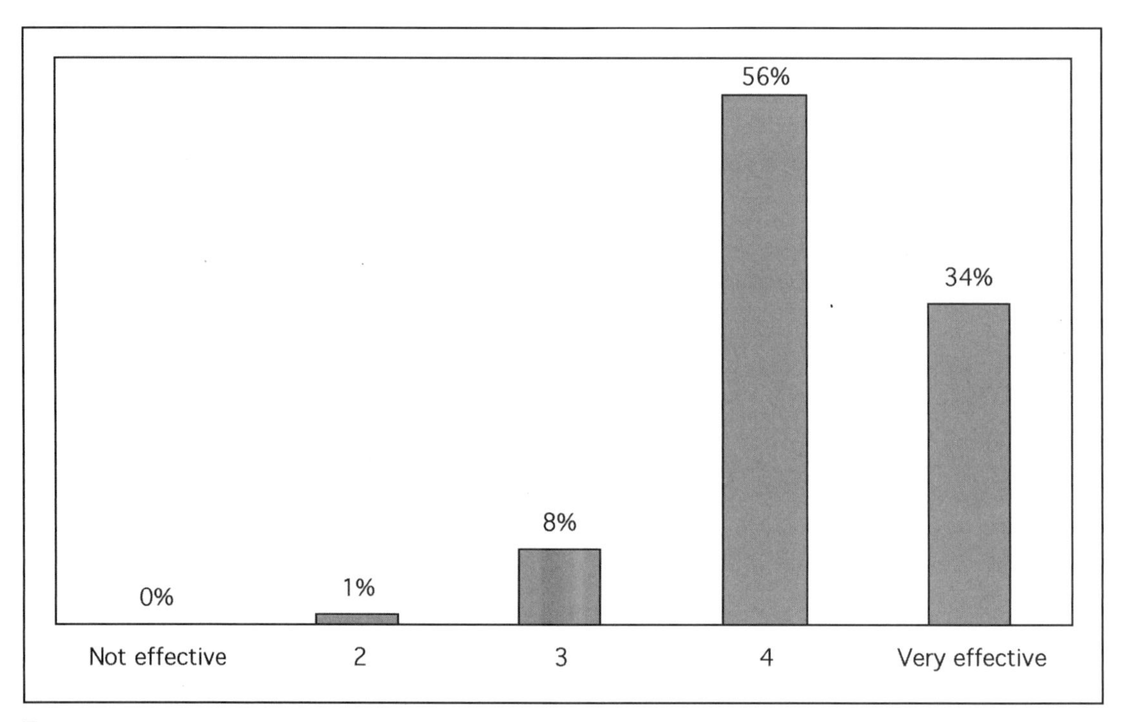

Figure 11.1. Percentages of 154 respondents who rated the effectiveness of the Lidcombe Program on a scale from 1 (*not effective*) to 5 (*very effective*).

was use of programs involving gradual increase in length and complexity of utterances (GILCU; Ryan, 1974) or extended length of utterance (ELU; Costello, 1983). A number of respondents indicated they used more than one other treatment. Interestingly, unsolicited comments from a number of respondents indicated that they include other treatment approaches within the Lidcombe Program.

Other unsolicited comments were also interesting. These comments were overwhelmingly positive about the program. Many respondents wanted more information about it and requested more professional development involving the program. However, scrutiny of the comments also indicated that there are some barriers to speech pathologists in Australia implementing the Lidcombe Program in the form in which it has been developed and researched. These mainly relate to workplace restrictions. For example, a number of respondents reported that they are unable to see clients once a week. This seemed to be particularly the case in rural areas, where it is known that clinicians may travel to satellite clinics and see clients infrequently (see Wilson, Lincoln, et al., 2002). Other respondents reported that they are restricted in the number of treatment hours they can allocate to each child in their caseload, or are required to see children in 6- to 8-week blocks. It seems unfortunate, then, that restrictions on service delivery imposed in the workplace—for whatever reasons—mean that Australian children who stutter may not always have access to a treatment that is widely researched and whose outcomes are supported by evidence.

Telehealth Delivery of the Lidcombe Program

As discussed previously, many Australian children and families live in remote or rural areas and cannot see a speech pathologist once each week, which is one of the requirements of

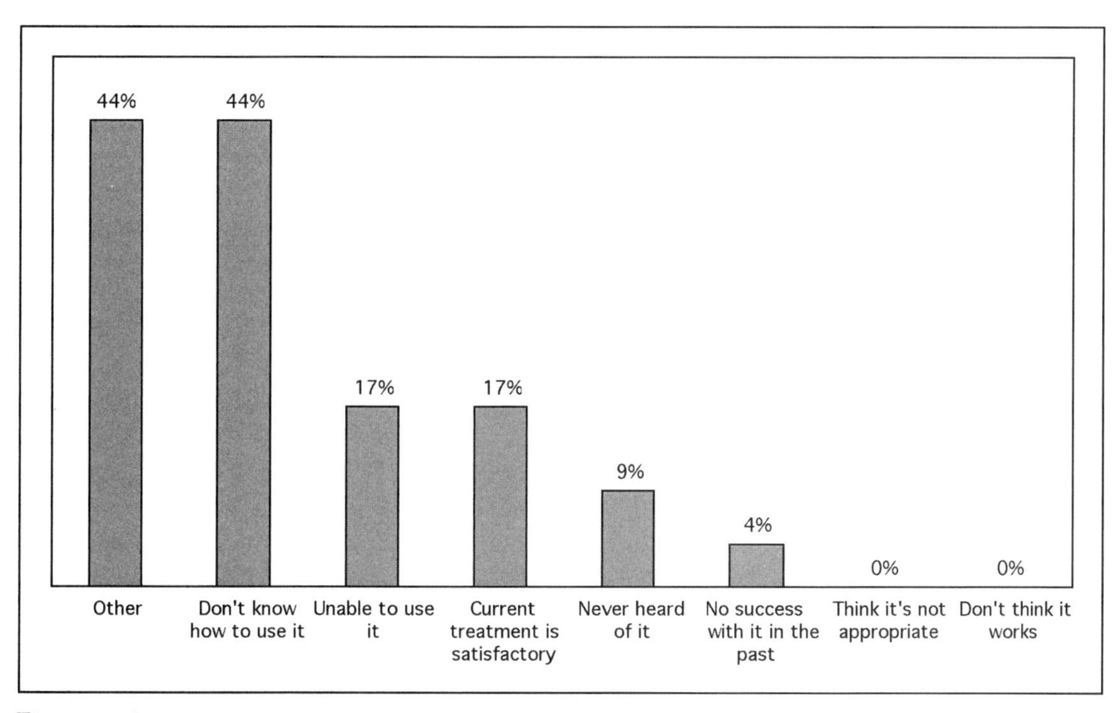

Figure 11.2. Reasons checked by 23 respondents for not using the Lidcombe Program.

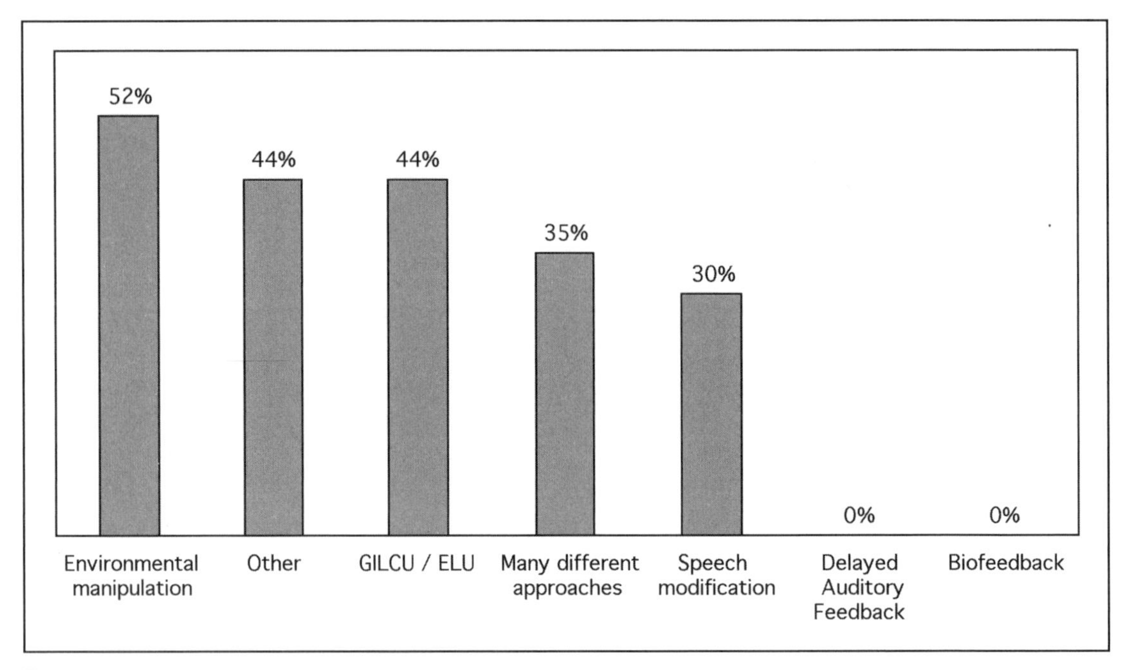

Figure 11.3. Other treatments used by 23 respondents who do not use the Lidcombe Program.

Stage 1 of the Lidcombe Program. Thus, a coordinated program of research is currently under way to investigate the effectiveness of delivering the Lidcombe Program via the use of telehealth. In Australia, the term *telehealth* refers to the use of information technologies and telecommunications (ITT) to support or deliver health services. The potential of ITT to improve access to services for rural and remote residents and other underserviced populations in Australia is well known (see Strong, Trickett, Titulaer, & Bhatia, 1998). A review of relevant Web sites at the time of writing indicated that a large number of telehealth projects are under way in Australia. Indeed, trials and research have demonstrated the viability and efficacy of a range of ITT options in a number of countries, in both health and education fields. As far as speech pathology services are concerned, in parts of Canada specialist consultations for stuttering are delivered by telehealth for clients and clinicians in remote areas (Kully & Langevin, 2000). This is of interest because, like Australia, Canada is a very large country with a relatively small population and large tracts of unsettled or sparsely populated land (see Chapter 13).

A pilot investigation into telehealth delivery of the Lidcombe Program in Australia was conducted from 1997 to 1998 by some of the authors of this chapter (Harrison, Wilson, & Onslow, 1999). In this case report, the mother of a British boy age 5 years 10 months who had been stuttering severely for 4 years delivered the Lidcombe Program in the child's natural environment, under the direction of the clinician in Australia. Phone contact occurred weekly, at least in the first part of treatment, and this was supplemented by the exchange of audiotapes and videotapes. The child's mother was instructed in how to deliver contingencies for stuttering and stutter-free speech and how to measure stuttering severity. She conducted daily treatment with the boy, progressing from treatment in structured to unstructured conversations as stipulated in the treatment manual. Indeed, the only essential feature of the program not implemented was the weekly clinic visits. Stage 1 was completed in 277 days (about 9 months), with 25 telephone consultations.

Stage 2 was also implemented as specified in the manual. Although performance criteria were not met on two occasions during Stage 2, the child went on to complete the maintenance component of the program successfully. The child's parents now report that the subject remains stutter-free. Stuttering measures—that is, percentage of syllables stuttered (%SS)—for the child made before and after Stage 1 are shown in Figure 11.4. These measures were made from recordings of the child speaking in a variety of everyday situations.

Subsequent case studies have confirmed that telehealth is a viable service delivery model for the Lidcombe Program. At the time of writing, researchers at the ASRC have obtained funding from the National Health and Medical Research Council of Australia to conduct a randomized controlled clinical trial of the delivery of the Lidcombe Program via telehealth. In this trial, preschool children who stutter are randomly allocated to either the treatment group or to a wait-list control group. Outcomes of the two groups will be compared over a number of months after randomization. Children in the wait-list group who continue to stutter will be offered treatment at a later date.

Conclusion

The genesis and subsequent development of the Lidcombe Program in Australia is outlined in Chapter 2. The purpose of this chapter, then, is to report on some issues that have arisen in Australia in relation to the implementation of the program, now that it has come of age. The first issue is that of the acceptance and usage of the Lidcombe Program by the wider clinical community in Australia. A survey of Australian speech pathologists indicated that the program has wide acceptance in Australia, being the treatment of choice for 87% of respondents who treat stuttering. Respondents were overwhelmingly positive in rating the effectiveness of the program and commented positively on other aspects of it. Respondents were considered to be a representative sample of speech pathologists in Australia.

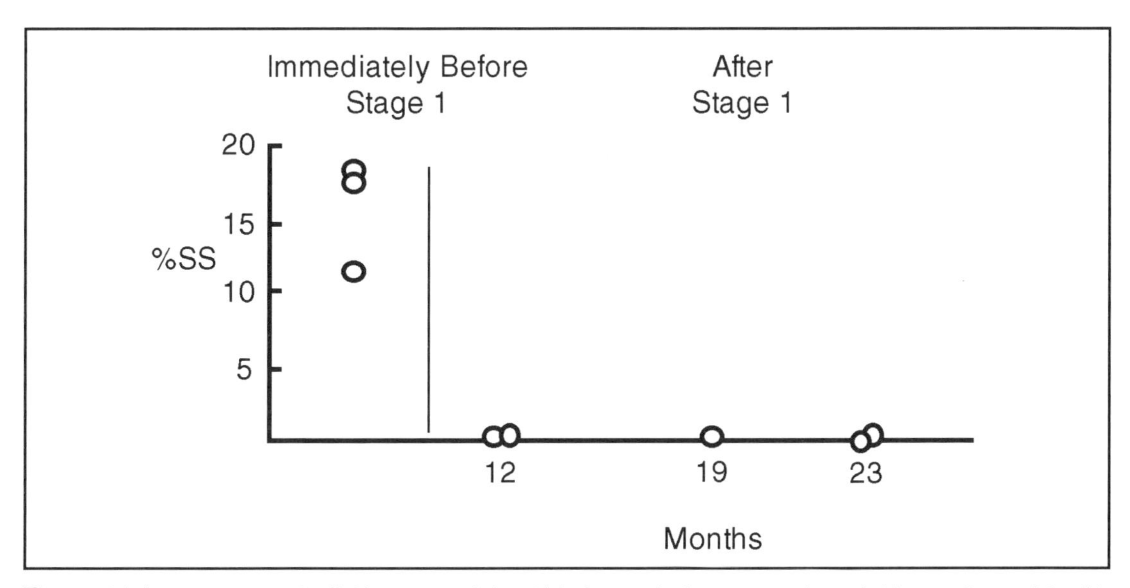

Figure 11.4. Percentage of syllables stuttered (%SS) before and after Stage 1 for a child treated via telehealth delivery of the Lidcombe Program (Harrison, Wilson, & Onslow, 1999).

It is clear, however, that the Lidcombe Program is not always implemented as it has been researched and as stipulated in the treatment manual. Clinicians do not always see children on a weekly basis and some clinicians reported combining the program with other treatment approaches. It should be said at this point that there is no evidence that the Lidcombe Program will have positive outcomes when essential components are omitted, when it is combined with other treatment approaches, or both.

The one exception to this is the preliminary evidence that the program may be effective when delivered with telehealth. The population of Australia is concentrated around certain coastal areas, particularly on the east coast. The inland of the continent is sparsely populated and the access of many isolated outback communities to health services, including speech pathology services, is very limited. As a response to this barrier to access to the Lidcombe Program, research into the delivery of the program through telehealth is currently under way. The program is particularly suited to such a service delivery model, as the treatment is actually delivered by parents in the child's natural environment. However, the telehealth model is not without hazards. Particular care needs to be taken to compensate for the lack of weekly visits where the clinician can establish, from direct observation, that the parent is implementing the program as directed and that the treatment is a positive experience for the child and parent. Nonetheless, the telehealth model holds promise of bringing a scientifically researched stuttering treatment to children for whom it would otherwise be inaccessible.

The goal of the developers of the Lidcombe Program is that every Australian child who starts to stutter will have access to the Lidcombe Program, if it is needed. The current systematic research into the program in Australia will hopefully go some way toward ensuring this.

References

Attanasio, M., Onslow, M., & Menzies, R. (1996). Australian and United States perspectives on stuttering in pre-school children. *Australian Journal of Human Communication Disorders, 24*, 55–61.

Cornick, S. (1996). *A description of service delivery to infants' school-age, language-impaired children*. Unpublished master's thesis, The University of Sydney.

Costello, J. M. (1983). Current behavioral treatments for stuttering. In D. Prins & R. J. Ingham (Eds.), *Treatment of stuttering in early childhood: Methods and issues* (pp. 69–112). San Diego: College-Hill Press.

Harrison, E., Wilson, L., & Onslow, M. (1999). Distance intervention for early stuttering with the Lidcombe Programme. *Advances in Speech–Language Pathology, 1*, 31–36.

Kully, D., & Langevin, M. (2000). Telehealth in stuttering treatment. *Journal of Fluency Disorders, 25*, 204.

Onslow, M., Costa, L., & Rue, S. (1990). Direct early intervention with stuttering: Some preliminary data. *Journal of Speech and Hearing Disorders, 55*, 405–416.

Packman, A., Onslow, M., & Menzies, R. (2000). Novel speech patterns and the control of stuttering. *Disability and Rehabilitation, 22*, 65–79.

Rousseau, I., Packman, A., Onslow, M., & Robinson, R. (2000). *The Lidcombe Program and Australian service delivery models: Survey of Australian speech pathol-ogists*. Poster presentation at the 2nd Asia Pacific Conference of Speech, Language and Hearing, Gold Coast, Australia.

Rousseau, I., Packman, A., Onslow, M., Dredge, R., & Harrison, E. (2002). Australian speech pathologists' use of the Lidcombe Program of early stuttering intervention. *ACQuiring Knowledge in Speech, Language and Hearing, 4*, 67–71.

Ryan, B. P. (1974). *Programmed therapy for stuttering in children and adults*. Springfield, IL: Thomas.

Strong, K., Trickett, P., Titulaer, I., & Bhatia, K. (1998). *Health in rural and remote Australia*. Canberra: Australian Institute of Health and Welfare.

Wilson, L., Lincoln, M., & Onslow, M. (2002). Availability, access, and quality of care: Inequities in rural speech pathology services and a model for redress. *Advances in Speech–Language Pathology, 4*, 9–22.

Wilson, L., Onslow, M., & Lincoln, M. (2002). *Treatment services for stuttering children in rural and remote areas*. Manuscript submitted for publication.

Chapter 12

The United Kingdom

Rosemarie Hayhow, Mary Kingston, and Rebeccah Ledzion

This chapter begins with a brief review of the approaches to stuttering therapy for adults and children used in the United Kingdom (UK) over the past 30 years. This material is presented as a context into which the Lidcombe Program was introduced in the mid-1990s. We describe that introduction, and we review Mary Kingston's audit of her own clinical efforts with the treatment, along with a national audit of the Lidcombe Program conducted by clinicians working during the 2 years after the initial UK training courses. Finally, clinical issues with the Lidcombe Program are explored from the perspectives of both clinicians and parents.

Historical Perspectives: The 1970s and 1980s

Therapy for Adults

Within the UK, some prominent clinicians who work with adults also work with children, so developments or changes with one age group tend to influence what happens with the other. Therefore, as a prelude to consideration of the treatment of early stuttering in the UK, this section reviews the work published by clinicians in that country who have long been influenced by the North American literature, and to a lesser extent by the behavioral therapies used in Australia.

In the 1970s, Irwin (1972) published the treatment effects of *easy stammering,* an adaptation of the work of Van Riper, with whom Irwin had studied in Iowa. At the same time, other direct methods for both adults and children were being explored in the context of group intensive therapy (e.g., Fawcus, 1970; Rustin, 1978; Watts, 1971). However, evaluation of intensive prolonged speech courses for adults, which were influenced by the work of Ingham and colleagues (e.g., Ingham, Andrews, & Winkler, 1972), showed poor results for some and poor long-term maintenance of therapy gains for others (Helps & Dalton, 1979). These results led to a renewed interest in the ideas behind the *stutter more fluently* therapies (e.g., Gregory, 1979; Van Riper, 1973) and enthusiasm for the work of Fransella (1972). Fransella's pioneering research using Personal Construct Theory (PCT; Kelly, 1955) showed that reductions in adult stuttering could be brought about by changes in thinking and feelings about speaking. Lasting change occurred when stuttering, fluency, or both were no longer the major filter through which all events and people were construed. A tension developed between behavioral or direct approaches and cognitive or indirect approaches, providing a stimulus for clinicians to develop their thinking and therapy procedures. One of the attractions of PCT for UK clinicians in the 1970s and early 1980s was that it viewed behavior, feeling, and thinking as inextricably linked. In addition, the notion of personal construct systems required clinicians to explore personal meanings and thus encouraged them to listen to and work with individuals rather than adopt the same treatment regime for all who stutter. This was more in sympathy with the eclectic approach of Van Riper than with the programmed behavioral approach of Ingham and colleagues.

Therapy for Children

In a self-help book for early stuttering, Irwin (1980) extended her easy stammering model to include children older than the age of 5 years. Treatment of younger children is "quite clear cut" (p. 51). She continues, "The parents and all members of the family, and all the people with whom the child associates must learn not to react to the stammering in any way whatsoever." Furthermore, she says, "If you do stop correcting him, that is not enough until you learn to stop looking anxious about it." This view of early stuttering is derived from Johnson's (1959) approach that stuttering will resolve if the parents remove the focus from speaking and reduce tensions for both themselves and the child (see Chapter 3). In a later book, Irwin (1988) concentrated on early stuttering, reiterating the same message of protecting the child from communicative and other pressures during the period of instability in fluency skills.

The availability of Irwin's books made her work influential. However, some clinicians looked beyond the stuttering literature at other models of change and development to find clinically useful ways of understanding early stuttering. In addition to PCT, Hayhow and Levy (1987) reported on ways in which their study of brief therapy and family therapy had influenced their work with children who stutter. Changes in the child's and parents' construing were found to have beneficial effects upon levels of stuttering and anxiety. The centrality of personal meanings within the PCT framework encouraged clinicians to try to understand the nature, significance, and effect of stuttering from the points of view of each family member. Brief therapy (Procter & Walker, 1987) assists parent and child to explore ways of managing stuttering and to abandon attempted solutions that are either maintaining stuttering or failing to reduce it. Such an approach encourages hypothesis forming and problem solving and helps to mitigate against attitudes and behaviors that reinforce stuttering.

However, Hayhow and Levy did not abandon all direct work. They suggested that, when required, direct therapy should be based on a gradual increase in length and complexity of utterances (Heinze & Johnson, 1985; Ryan & Van Kirk, 1978) so that the child could build upon existing fluency skills. They recommended that, during clinic visits, the therapist model new home tasks, which the parent then tried out in the session. Therapist feedback for the parent ensured that the activities were done in the way intended. Generalization was encouraged by systematically increasing the demands and pressures within clinic or home-based sessions so that they became more and more like everyday situations.

Historical Perspectives: The 1990s

The work described so far shows how stuttering therapy was developing in the UK during the 1970s and 1980s. The 1990s saw the publication in the UK of two more books, both resulting from many years of clinical experience, and both written by well-respected teams of clinicians who had taught their respective approaches extensively, at undergraduate and postgraduate levels. The first book, by Stewart and Turnbull (1995), describes an approach that is influenced by the work of Van Riper (1973, 1990) and by the Demands and Capacities model (Starkweather & Gottwald, 1990). The second book, by Rustin, Botterill, and

Kelman (1996), describes the interaction approach developed by the Michael Palin Centre for Stammering Children.

Stewart and Turnbull

Stewart and Turnbull, like Irwin (1988), have written self-help books for both parents and children who stutter (Stewart & Turnbull, 1995, 1996). Also like Irwin, they believe in protecting the child from unhelpful demands, but in addition consider developing the child's capacities. They describe the Demands and Capacities model, integrating this with other models and ideas for early dysfluency, borderline and confirmed stuttering. With young children there is often an initial emphasis on indirect work, but the notion of increasing the child's capacities allows for direct work when appropriate. Stewart and Turnbull (1995) recommend that the clinician demonstrates for the parents a communicative style that facilitates fluency and also provides them with information and ideas about how to modify the child's speaking environment. By identifying fluency disrupters and fluency enhancers, the parents become more able to influence their child's level of stuttering. The aim of therapy with children in the early dysfluency stage is to ensure that the child does not develop maladaptive ways of coping. The aim for those who are showing borderline stuttering is that they should respond to their "non-fluencies as lags and reconstrue themselves positively, irrespective of their speech" (p. 54).

The Michael Palin Centre

Another important influence on work with early stuttering in the UK has been the Michael Palin Centre. Clinicians at this center have been influential not only through the development of their family interaction therapy and intensive courses (Rustin, 1978; Rustin et al., 1996; Rustin, Cook, & Spence, 1995), but by establishing the Oxford Dysfluency Conference and arranging many short courses and workshops run by visiting North American specialists, such as Bruce Ryan, Hugo Gregory, Edward Conture, and Barry Guitar. These learning opportunities demystified the work of colleagues across the Atlantic and helped many clinicians feel more confident in their work with children who stutter. The family interaction therapy of Rustin et al. (1996) aims to modify those parental behaviors that are thought to influence the child's level of stuttering. There is a prescribed assessment procedure and a 6-week course of therapy for the child and both parents, followed by a period of consolidation and review. Direct work is considered only when a course of therapy and period of consolidation have failed to produce adequate change in the child's speech. The Michael Palin Centre team members advocate their adaptation of a cognitive behavioral approach (Meyers & Woodford, 1992), whereby the child is taught the concepts of slow versus fast, smooth versus bumpy, and hard versus easy. These concepts are then related to speaking, and the child imitates the therapist's model of slow, smooth, and easy speech, which the therapist reinforces. Home practice aids transfer and the child develops an understanding of "the underlying concepts which are used to modify dysfluency, and is able to implement changes based on that awareness" (p. 133). Although relatively few preschool children require such direct therapy, it is claimed that this approach has been successful.

Expectation of Therapy Outcome

Van Riper has been a consistent influence in the UK over the past 30 years. In one of his last writings about stuttering (Van Riper, 1990), he discussed stuttering as a "neuromuscular disorder whose core consists of tiny lags and disruptions in the timing of the complicated movements required for speech" (p. 317). He believed that for some, these lags will continue for life, which raised questions about what might constitute a realistic outcome for young clients. Van Riper suggested that some individuals outgrow their stuttering either because they do not react to the lags with repetitions of syllables or prolongations of sounds, or that with maturation the lags gradually disappear. He suggested that those who learn to struggle and avoid in response to these lags will continue to do so. Therefore, therapy should help the person to accept that the lags will always be there and to establish a form of easy stuttering.

Although achievable outcomes were often not defined in the UK literature, there was probably a general agreement with Van Riper's beliefs that therapy should aim to reduce speech-related anxiety and fear. The reduced anxiety and fear then lead to reduced intensity and, therefore, frequency of stuttering. Evidence that such therapy was more effective at reducing anxiety than stuttering was reported in an extensive audit of therapy services for more than 200 children who stutter in Northern Ireland (Watson, Preston, & Riches, 1996). The audit showed that 68% of respondents felt that therapy led to reductions in child or parent anxiety, 28% of parents felt better able to deal with the problem, 3% felt their child's confidence had improved, but only 1% reported improvement in fluency. The audit arose from dissatisfaction with the services for children who stutter, and the results supported the clinicians' beliefs that changes were needed both to the structure of services and to therapy procedures.

Themes and Issues in the Treatment of Early Stuttering in the United Kingdom

Some themes have emerged from published work in the UK during the past 30 years. First, clinicians avoid talking about the elimination of stuttering because of the belief that it is an unachievable goal for some children. It is feared that the subsequent sense of failure and possible negative attitudes toward the remaining stuttering are harmful because they are among those factors identified by adult clients and the literature as being influential in increasing the handicapping aspects of stuttering. Second, tensions between change in behavior versus change in attitudes and direct versus indirect approaches are apparent, but there is little research evidence to help clinicians select the best therapy approach for a particular child. Finally, clinicians favor an eclectic approach, resisting the use of one theoretical model or program of therapy in preference for combining, from a variety of sources, the approaches and activities that they believe to be appropriate to individual families.

Historically, UK clinicians have had to rely on expert opinion from colleagues at home. However, the need for hard evidence of efficacy has become more pressing as changes have occurred within the National Health Service. It is no longer enough to know that a particular approach has been found to be helpful within a particular context. We need much more specific therapy outcomes and, ideally, these need to be linked in clear ways to particular therapy activities or options.

Discussion with clinicians at study days and conferences revealed a growing concern about the small but too large group of children who did not respond to indirect therapy. Fawcus (1995) voiced this concern: "In advocating an indirect approach in the management of early stuttering and working only through the parents, clinicians have in the past not always taken sufficient account of the child's awareness of his own disfluent speech" (p. 6). Some clinicians wanted to develop skills in safe and effective direct work that did not require the child to learn some modified speech pattern or speech techniques. In addition, there was research (e.g., Bernstein Ratner, 1992; Weiss & Zebrowski, 1992) that brought into question some of the assumptions that underlie the indirect approaches described previously. This has affected clinicians' confidence in suggesting changes in parental communication behavior in the absence of hard evidence showing that it is beneficial for the child.

The Introduction of the Lidcombe Program in the United Kingdom

The British Stammering Association (BSA) became aware of the Lidcombe Program through contact with the parents of a child who stuttered who were unable to procure treatment in their local area (Harrison, Wilson, & Onslow, 1999). They received distance intervention from the team in Sydney with good results. The BSA then arranged for Mark Onslow to give a presentation about the Lidcombe Program at St. Thomas' Hospital in London at the end of 1995. Subsequently, the BSA arranged a lecture tour of universities, hospitals, and clinics across Scotland, Ireland, England, and the Channel Islands in 1996. This tour stimulated a lively debate in both the professional literature and the press. Clinicians were interested in, and at times, critical of, the Lidcombe approach, and parents wanted to know more. The UK history of indirect therapy meant that many clinicians were initially hostile to the approach, although some wished to learn more about this reportedly safe and effective way of working directly on the young child's speech.

Subsequently, we attended a 2-week intensive Lidcombe Program training period in Sydney and, after returning to the UK, used the program in our specialist stuttering clinics. During the next 6 months, it became apparent that the treatment was able to be replicated by clinicians across the world from Lidcombe, Australia, and an increasing number of UK clinicians requested training. January 1998 saw the beginning of UK-based training courses. The first three courses were run by Sue O'Brian from the Australian Stuttering Research Centre, and since then we have continued with training in the UK and Ireland. We present some of the issues that have emerged during these courses and describe the ongoing supports that have developed as a result of clinicians' needs to develop their skills with the treatment over time.

Initial Concerns About the Lidcombe Program

Earlier in the chapter we discussed how correction was specifically identified by Irwin (1972) as a parental behavior considered instrumental in the maintenance of stuttering. It was therefore not surprising that therapists were concerned to find that requests for self-correction is used in the Lidcombe Program. Irwin's warnings against correction stemmed from the view of early stuttering as a variant of normal nonfluency, a view shared by Stewart (1996), who referred to the dangers of correcting a "normal developmental sequence" (p. 4). In the same article, Stewart warned that correction may undermine the child and lead to a construction of self as "stammerer" and hence make the problem more severe.

Another key issue in the debate about the Lidcombe Program concerned the nature of early stuttering. Is it, as Onslow, O'Brian, and Harrison (1997) claim, "a relatively simple, physical speech dysfunction" (p. 237) or a complex disorder arising from the interaction of multiple variables? Both Stewart (1996) and Rustin and Cook (1997) took the latter view, in agreement with contemporary research and thinking at the time in the United States, UK, and Europe. Onslow et al. (1997) argued that multifactorial symptomatology does not necessarily mean a multifactorial cause. Either way, this still leaves open the question of whether a complex problem can be alleviated by a conceptually simple treatment. Is it the case, as Stewart suggests, that a complex problem cannot be managed by changing one factor among the many? Or is it possible that a change in one element of the problem can lead to changes in the problem overall? It could be argued that this latter view underlies the indirect therapy approaches, in which changes in parental behavior are thought to lead ultimately to changes in the child's speech.

Another issue was whether the Australian team had sufficient data to support their claims. Published data supporting the program reported on far fewer cases than the 500-plus reportedly treated at the Lidcombe and Bankstown clinics at the time (Onslow & Harrison, 1995), hence raising questions concerning the outcomes for the unpublished children. Rustin and Cook (1997) point out that long-term results indicate (Lincoln & Onslow, 1997) that at least 29% of parents were aware of their children stuttering again sometime between 1 and 3 years after the completion of treatment.

Concern was also expressed about the demands made upon parents in this treatment as outlined by Onslow and Harrison (1995). Many therapists in the UK thought that parents would find such demands difficult and possibly in conflict with their view of their parental role. In addition, the centrality of the parents' role in the Lidcombe Program suggested to some UK therapists that factors other than response-contingent stimulation could be having a treatment effect.

This discussion of concerns about the Lidcombe Program when it was first widely publicized in the UK might give the impression that no one would find it a viable treatment option. However, there were clinicians who wanted a safe and effective way to work directly with young children who stutter, a way that did not impose an artificially slow speech pattern or require conscious modification of sound production. For some more experienced clinicians, the issue was not so much whether the Lidcombe Program worked as claimed for all children but rather whether it might be an appropriate and effective treatment for some; in particular, for those children who continue to stutter in spite of a supportive and facilitating home environment and whose distress at their stuttering was becoming disabling.

Rosemarie Hayhow and Mary Kingston were two therapists with many years of experience, both working in specialist posts with children and adults who stutter. A 1-day workshop run by Onslow and O'Brian in Bristol, England, had given Hayhow enough of an understanding to use the program with three children, all of whom did extremely well, which prompted a desire for more training. Rebecca Ledzion, although working in London, had trained in Australia and so was familiar with the Lidcombe Program. However, the high profile of the treatment in the UK prompted her to combine a trip home to Australia with a refresher course. After much organization, the three met for the first time on the first day of the 2-week course in Sydney. The course comprised seminars, presentations, and clinical observation of different clinicians working with children at different stages in treatment. The 2 weeks were stimulating, with many opportunities for discussion and sharing of views. On our return to England, the three of us were able to support each other as we integrated the Lidcombe Program into our clinical practice. Over the next few months, many clinicians expressed an interest in the program, so in early 1998 three training courses were held, one in each of our respective National Health Service Trusts. Sue O'Brian came from Australia to run the courses. Thus the UK-based training started.

Training in the Lidcombe Program Within the UK and Ireland

At the time of writing, 20 *basic training* courses have occurred since January 1998, with approximately 280 clinicians attending. Most courses run for 5 or 6 days, comprising 3 days of theory and 1 day of observation, with at least 1 follow-up day around 6 months. Some clinicians favor 2 follow-up days, with the final meeting about 1 year after the initial course.

Further *continuing training* days (Lidcombe Link Days) are held around the country so clinicians can continue to meet and share their successes and problems. Occasionally, Mark Onslow has been able to attend these days, thus allowing for more formal updating of Australian research and clinical practice.

Mary Kingston established and produces the *Lidcombe News*, which is a newsletter with three editions a year. Subscriptions have risen in line with the increasing numbers of speech–language therapists trained to use the Lidcombe Program, from 32 at initial subscription in May 1998 to 165 in April 2001. The numbers subscribing give an indication of how many clinicians use the program; at the time of writing there are currently 216 clinicians on the directory of trained clinicians. However, few clinicians in Ireland subscribe to the newsletter, even though we are informed that the approach is popular and we are regularly approached to run more courses.

Studies of Children Treated with the Lidcombe Program in the United Kingdom

Two studies provide information on children treated with the Lidcombe Program in the UK. First, an audit (Lane & Kingston, 2000), carried out in Norfolk between May 1997 and July 1999, detailed 52 families who had received the Lidcombe Program. Second, a nationwide audit of cases seen between January 1998 and December 1999 comprised data from 30 clinicians on 247 children (Hayhow & Enderby, 2001a, 2001b). A review of these studies helps to address some of the areas of concern that were identified earlier in the chapter. One initial aim of the audits was to collate data on short-term outcome to see if UK results were similar to those achieved by the Australian team. It was found that the children treated in Norwich (Kingston, 1999) took the same median number of clinic visits (i.e., 11) to reach Stage 2 as reported by the Australian team (Jones, Onslow, Harrison, & Packman, 2000). The national audit reported a median of 9 clinic visits (Hayhow & Enderby, 2001a).

A parent questionnaire was designed specifically to investigate the previously identified areas of concern. The first version was piloted in Norfolk, Bristol, and London on cases we had treated (Hayhow, Enderby, & Kingston, 2000). The final questionnaire was given to 147 parents, and 106 (72%) were returned. The parents reported favorable treatment outcomes for their children, with 71% rarely or never stuttering. There was no evidence that this was the result of the children's talking less or being overanxious not to stutter. In fact, 75% of parents felt their child had become "much" or "a little" more confident. There was no change in perceived confidence levels in 24% of the children, with some parents commenting that stuttering had never affected their child's confidence. A majority of 94% "disagreed" or "mostly disagreed" that therapy was disruptive for the rest of the family, and 93% agreed that they were "pleased to be able to help their child themselves." In written responses some parents (41%) mentioned problems in organization and time. However, many of these also commented that the time and planning were worthwhile once they saw the progress that their child was making. Only 3 parents were not sure that they would recommend the approach to other parents.

These studies showed that the short-term results obtained in the UK with the Lidcombe Program are comparable to those cited by Onslow and colleagues. Further research is required to determine the long-term results.

Parents in the UK do not report that the treatment demands too much of them and they do not see evidence of any harmful side effects from aiming to eliminate stuttering. The high response rate from parents shows their willingness to be involved in evaluation studies, so a modified questionnaire is being developed that UK clinicians can use routinely as part of their outcome measures.

Clinical Issues

Since the systematic introduction of the Lidcombe Program to the UK in May 1997, and the start of training courses in January 1998, two further initiatives have allowed us to gather evidence about clinical issues arising from the changes in our thinking required by the program. The *Lidcombe News*, previously mentioned, has been a vehicle for chronicling views of clinicians, parents, and children alike, and the institution of the Lidcombe Link Days around the country has enabled clinicians to meet to air problems and successes, and to discuss issues arising from the new approach. Information gained from the *Lidcombe News* and Lidcombe Link Days suggests that the beliefs and traditions about stuttering that parents and clinicians bring with them to treatment have had an effect on the way the program is carried out in the UK. This has made our experience of it different from that in Australia, where changes in stuttering behavior rather than in attitudes toward stuttering have been the primary focus of stuttering treatment for preschool children.

The indirect treatment carried out in this country with young children, described earlier in the chapter, was based on the idea that stuttering is a highly complex condition consisting of many contributing factors that serve to precipitate and perpetuate the problem. Environmental and interactive pressures on the child in such an approach were therefore areas of focus for the clinician and the parents. The Lidcombe Program, with its central emphasis on the child's speech, was viewed as simplistic for failing to take into account these wider issues. This narrower focus is an issue for both clinicians and parents. One mother wrote in the *Lidcombe News* (May 1999, p. 8), "I think we were initially a bit sceptical about whether it would work because it sounds so simple." Another parent, delighted at the ultimate success of the program with her child, commented, "It is hard to believe that such a simple technique can have such amazing results" (*Lidcombe News*, May 2001, p. 4). In the early stages, therefore, parents may have to be persuaded that the program is worth a try. Some parents, after using the program, have admitted to us that initially they thought such an approach would never work.

The overarching clinical consideration in this country, therefore, has been whether an indirect approach or a direct speech-focused form of treatment is the most effective with young children who stutter. However, although indirect methods have in recent history been preferred in the UK, we believe that the majority of clinicians in this country are neither convinced they are the only approach nor averse to direct methods per se. Rather, the issue arose because, before the Lidcombe Program arrived, there was a dearth of demonstrably safe and effective treatments available to us—certainly ones that did not impose a modified speech pattern upon the young child. This is borne out by the results of a survey conducted by Onslow and O'Brian in the UK in the summer of 1996 ("Onslow Tour," 1996, p. 4), in which 75% of clinicians responded "yes" to the question about whether they would consider using the direct approach of the Lidcombe Program, whereas 23% responded "not sure" and only 2% said "no."

Despite an openness to direct methods, many clinicians have had to readjust the ways they have looked at and understood stuttering. A clinician from Birmingham wrote, "As a Specialist in Fluency Disorders I was unprepared for how the Lidcombe would shake my beliefs and expectations about stammering" (*Lidcombe News*, May 2000, p. 9). A clinician from Ireland commented that the Lidcombe Program is "quite strong stuff" for those used to an "arms length" therapy model (*Lidcombe News*, January 2001, p. 7).

The direct approach and the centrality of feedback on the child's speech in the Lidcombe Program has conflicted with the prevailing belief among many clinicians and parents that it is safest not to make an issue of stuttering with the child. "We were concerned that by drawing attention to it and expecting her to control it we could end up destroying her confidence and worsening her stuttering," wrote one parent (*Lidcombe News*, May 1998, p. 5). Having embarked on the treatment, another parent wrote,

> I didn't have too much difficulty in giving praise for smooth talking, however I found it much harder (when the child's speech was reasonably fluent) to correct a poorly spoken word. I found that I hesitated to say anything and the moment passed without correction. (*Lidcombe News*, May 1999, p. 8)

Once the issue of feedback is overcome, however, a sense of relief is evident from parents, one of whom wrote,

> This was like a breath of fresh air to us, at long last we could talk to (the child) about the stutter, actively encourage her to overcome it and share in her enjoyment as she progressed from a daily marking of 7 down to her first 1 marking, meaning no stutters for a whole day. (*Lidcombe News*, September 1998, p. 4)

As parental verbal contingencies are so vital to the success of the Lidcombe Program, questions have been raised about implementation of the program when the parents themselves stutter. Concerns that these parents will be unable to offer smooth models and that a mixed message is being given by the parents who are stuttering themselves and yet are asking for stutter-free speech, have been seen by some as a potential problem for the child. Another concern is that the stuttering parents are receiving a negative message about themselves, trying as they are to live with and accept their own stutter, and yet attempting to eliminate that of their child by praising stutter-free speech. However, in our experience, this has not held treatment back or caused difficulties for child or parent. Indeed, the opposite experience has been the case. As one parent wrote,

> Within a few months H's speech had greatly improved with her smooth talking, also I couldn't believe the confidence in both of us. Even family members commented on how well *both* our speeches had improved! (*Lidcombe News*, September 1998, p. 5)

A clinician from Swindon, also broaching this issue, wrote in the *Lidcombe News* (September 2000, p. 11),

> One child happily started commenting on his mum's talking as well! This was very helpful, as he would say when his mum was smooth.

This aided his own self-evaluation and progress toward stutter-free speech. Far from feeling negative about themselves, therefore, it is our experience that the self-esteem of stuttering parents is raised by the experience of helping their child overcome difficulties with speaking.

Further issues involving use of the Lidcombe Program center on the concerns for the child if treatment fails to eliminate stuttering. The worry is that the child who continues to stutter will be left with a negative self-image as a result of believing that bumpy speech is "bad." Parents are aware that stuttering can cause problems in the way children feel about themselves, and some are fearful for their children's social and personal well-being. In Kingston's (1999) audit, the main concerns of parents' prior to treatment had to do with school and bullying, frustration, and upset because of the stuttering behavior, other children not listening to them, and a loss of confidence. A parent sums this up in the newsletter:

> Our real fear was that because of his stammering, he might be teased or bullied, resulting in lack of confidence and low self-esteem. (*Lidcombe News*, September 1999, p. 4)

Given these anxieties, some parents and clinicians are fearful of giving the message that it is not good to stutter, which is implicit in the praise given to stutter-free speech in the Lidcombe Program. In particular, they are concerned that if a child has to live with stuttering for life, this message may put him or her at risk of developing avoidance behaviors and negative attitudes. Work will then have to be done through counseling, and modification therapies (Sheehan, 1986; Van Riper, 1973), to foster an open and accepting attitude toward stuttering.

It is essential, therefore, when teaching the Lidcombe Program to explain that requests for the child to self-correct stuttering are neutral rather than critical. Success in correcting the stuttering is undoubtedly pleasing to the child, but this need not necessarily mean that when children stutter they will feel badly about it.

The historical indirect methods of treatment in the UK have focused on environmental and interactional pressures to account for perpetuating stuttering in the young child, and parents may also see these as important factors. One mother wrote,

> Three years ago I spent an agonising summer holiday feeling unable to tell him off because I believed that it would make him stammer more . . . at this stage we were convinced that his stammer would become worse if he knew that we were worried about his speech. (*Lidcombe News*, January 2001, p. 5)

The idea that a child's speech system is vulnerable to a multiplicity of factors has become a clinical issue in the implementation of the Lidcombe Program in the UK. When fluctuations in the child's stuttering behavior are noted, the temptation is to fall back on the pressures of situations or environmental explanations from previous treatment approaches to account for the changes. Although there may well be some truth in them, they are not necessarily clinically useful in determining the next step in the treatment. Parents in the UK, therefore, may need help to use their clinical and problem-solving skills, learning to deal actively with increases in stuttering behavior, or lack of progress, with the methods they have been taught, rather than looking for environmental causes and remedies. However, once parents have learned to use the treatment, the resulting sense of empowerment is evident, both from the aforementioned audits and from the *Lidcombe News* perspectives. One parent wrote,

> I just kept a closer eye on his speech when special things happened like changing school, and Christmas or any other occasions which took him out of his regular routine because before this was when his speech was at its worst. (*Lidcombe News*, May 2001, p. 5)

Issues Arising from Lidcombe Link Days

The clinical issues discussed above are often raised at Lidcombe Link Days around the country, during which clinicians trained in the Lidcombe Program meet for purposes of continuing education. The debate about the "good to speak fluently and bad to stutter" message when a child is unsuccessful with the program continues, largely unresolved. Some clinicians, however, feel that having a top age for administering the program goes some way toward providing a solution, though what age this might be continues to be discussed. Alternatively, others believe we should be looking at the type of stuttering and the child's ability to correct it easily rather than at age levels.

Also unresolved is the appropriate therapy format for children with other conditions that affect speech, such as dyspraxia, Down syndrome, and a diagnosis of autistic spectrum disorder. Some clinicians feel that the program is not appropriate in such circumstances. As they do with older children who find it difficult to control their stuttering, these clinicians may use a combination of approaches rather than only the Lidcombe Program.

The clinical issues discussed previously have centered around the beliefs and views that parents and clinicians have brought to therapy. However, there are other areas of concern that clinicians have debated at the Lidcombe Link Days, which also need discussing. In particular, children from areas of the country with a considerable non–English speaking population bring their own challenges in implementing the Lidcombe Program. In a multiracial area of London, trained bilingual coworkers have been used effectively to overcome the language barrier, although the time taken to reach Stage 2 is longer (*Lidcombe News*, September 1999, p. 6).

Increasingly in the UK, we have families where both parents are working, or where working single parents have the care of the stuttering child. As the program is parent based, difficulties may therefore arise in carrying out the treatment. Ways around this time issue have been discussed at Link Days, centering on how the treatment load may be shared among other family members or caregivers who are able to come to the clinics. Parents can also obtain help from schools and nurseries, although this is recommended only if the clinician is able personally to train the professional involved.

Another important issue raised at Lidcombe Link Days has to do with clinician training, and the recognition that this needs to be rigorous if the program is to be safe and effective. There have been instances in the UK where those who have attended the recognized workshops have offered much reduced training to their colleagues and expected them to conduct the program. These colleagues not only are inadequately trained but also fall outside the support networks offered in this country, which are much valued by new trainees, for the sharing of expertise and good practice. We are often contacted by anxious parents who have had experience with those who have inadequate training. In these situations, we have found that elements of the program, usually the measurement components (see Chapter 5), are left out or misunderstood, and that the parent has not been trained adequately in the presentation of verbal contingencies. We strongly recommend that no clinician attempt to use the Lidcombe Program without attending comprehensive training.

Another issue related to training is the problem of clinical referral when families move out of an area with a Lidcombe clinician to one where the treatment is of a different kind. As more clinicians are trained, this may resolve. For now, however, the database of trainees that has been built up as part of the *Lidcombe News* can help families to find the nearest Lidcombe-trained clinician.

Finally, a service delivery issue arises from the need for regular clinic visits until the child's stuttering meets program criteria because, in some National Health Service Trusts, services are restricted to 6-week blocks of therapy. The inevitable variability in time taken to reach Stage 2 makes successful implementation of the program problematic. Where such restrictions exist, we suggest that the program not be introduced until this time issue is resolved with individual managers.

References

Bernstein Ratner, N. (1992). Measurable outcomes of instructions to modify normal parent–child verbal interactions: Implications for indirect stuttering therapy. *Journal of Speech and Hearing Research, 35*, 14–20.

Fawcus, M. (1970). Intensive treatment and group therapy for the child and adult stammerer. *British Journal of Disorders of Communication, 5*, 59–65.

Fawcus, M. (Ed.). (1995). *Stuttering: From theory to practice*. London: Whurr Publishers.

Fransella, F. (1972). *Personal change and reconstruction*. London: Academic Press.

Gregory, H. (1979). *Controversies about stuttering therapy*. Baltimore: University Park Press.

Harrison, E., Wilson, L., & Onslow, M. (1999). Distance intervention for early stuttering with the Lidcombe Programme. *Advances in Speech–Language Pathology, 1*, 31–36.

Hayhow, R., & Enderby, P. (2001a). *An audit of speech and language therapists' use of the Lidcombe Program*. Unpublished manuscript, Speech and Language Therapy Research Unit, Frenchay Hospital, Bristol, UK.

Hayhow, R., & Enderby, P. (2001b). *Parents' perceptions of the Lidcombe Program*. Unpublished manuscript, Speech and Language Therapy Research Unit, Frenchay Hospital, Bristol, UK.

Hayhow, R., Enderby, P., & Kingston, M. (2000). Parental satisfaction with stammering therapy: The development of a questionnaire. In H. G. Bosshardt, J. S. Yaruss, & H. F. M. Peters (Eds.), *Fluency disorders: Theory, research, treatment and self-help. Proceedings of the Third World Congress of Fluency Disorders* (pp. 322–325). Nyborg, Denmark: Nijmegen University Press.

Hayhow, R., & Levy, C. (1987). *Working with stuttering: A personal construct therapy approach*. Bicester, UK: Winslow Press.

Heinze, B., & Johnson, K. (1985). *Easy does it: Fluency activities for young children*. East Moline, IL: Lingui-Systems.

Helps, R., & Dalton, P. (1979). The effectiveness of an intensive group therapy programme for adult stammerers. *British Journal of Disorders of Communication, 14*, 17–30.

Ingham, R., Andrews, G., & Winkler, R. (1972). Stuttering: A comparative evaluation of the short term effectiveness of four treatment techniques. *Journal of Communication Disorders, 5*, 91–117.

Irwin, A. (1972). The treatment and results of "easy-stammering." *British Journal of Disorders of Communication, 7*, 151–156.

Irwin, A. (1980). *Stammering: Practical help for all ages*. Harmondsworth, UK: Penguin Books.

Irwin, A. (1988). *Stammering in young children*. Wellingborough, UK: Thorsons Publishing.

Johnson, W. (1959). *The onset of stuttering*. Minneapolis: University of Minnesota Press.

Jones, M., Onslow, M., Harrison, E., & Packman, A. (2000). Treating stuttering in young children: Predicting treatment time in the Lidcombe Program. *Journal of Speech, Language, and Hearing Research, 43*, 1440–1450.

Kelly, G. (1955). *The psychology of personal constructs* (Vols. 1 and 2). New York: Norton.

Kingston, M. (1999, December). Is stuttering a motor speech problem? *Bulletin of the Royal College of Speech & Language Therapists*, pp. 9–11.

Lane, J., & Kingston, M. (2000). *Words*. Unpublished manuscript.

Lincoln, M., & Onslow, M. (1997). Long-term outcome of an early intervention for stuttering. *American Journal of Speech–Language Pathology, 6*, 51–58.

Meyers, S., & Woodford, L. L. (1992). *The fluency development system for young children*. Buffalo, NY: United Educational Services.

Onslow, M., & Harrison, E. (1995). The Lidcombe Programme for early stuttering intervention. *Speaking Out, 16*(3), 4–5.

Onslow, M., O'Brian, S., & Harrison, E. (1997). The Lidcombe Program of early stuttering intervention: Methods and issues. *European Journal of Disorders of Communication, 32*, 231–250.

Onslow tour stimulates therapist debate [Editorial]. (1996). *Speaking Out, 17*(2).

Procter, H., & Walker, G. (1987). Brief therapy. In E. Street (Ed.), *Family therapy in Britain* (pp. 127–149). New York: Harper & Row.

Rustin, L. (1978). An intensive group programme for adolescent stammerers. *British Journal of Disorders of Communication, 13*, 85–92.

Rustin, L., Botterill, W., & Kelman, E. (1996). *Assessment and therapy for young disfluent children: Family interaction*. London: Whurr Publishers.

Rustin, L., & Cook, F. (1997). Commentary on the Lidcombe Program of early stuttering intervention. *European Journal of Disorders of Communication, 32*, 250–258.

Rustin, L., Cook, F., & Spence, R. (1995). *The management of stuttering in adolescence*. London: Whurr Publishers.

Ryan, B., & Van Kirk, B. (1978). *Monterey Fluency Program*. Palo Alto, CA: Monterey Learning Systems.

Sheehan, J. (1986). Theory and treatment of stuttering as an approach–avoidance conflict. In G. G. Shames & H. Rubin (Eds.), *Stuttering then and now* (pp. 187–200). Columbus, OH: Merrill.

Starkweather, C. W., & Gottwald, S. (1990). The demands capacities model II: Clinical applications. *Journal of Fluency Disorders, 15*, 143–157.

Stewart, T. (1996). A critique of the Lidcombe Programme for children who stammer. *Speaking Out, 17*, p. 4.

Stewart, T., & Turnbull, J. (1995). *Working with dysfluent children*. Bicester, UK: Winslow Press.

Stewart, T., & Turnbull, J. (1996). *Helping children cope with stammering*. London: Sheldon Press.

Van Riper, C. (1973). *The treatment of stuttering*. Englewood Cliffs, NJ: Prentice Hall.

Van Riper, C. (1990). Final thoughts about stuttering. *Journal of Fluency Disorders, 15*, 317–318.

Watson, D., Preston, B., & Riches, J. (1996). *An audit of service provision for children and adults with fluency disorders in Northern Ireland*. Unpublished manuscript.

Watts, F. (1971). The treatment of stammering by the intensive practice of fluent speech. *British Journal of Disorders of Communication, 6*, 144–147.

Weiss, A., & Zebrowski, P. (1992). Disfluencies in the conversations of young children who stutter: Some answers about questions. *Journal of Speech and Hearing Research, 35*, 1230–1238.

Chapter 13

Canada

Rosalee Shenker and JoAnne Wilding

The Lidcombe Program was virtually unheard of in Canada prior to 1997. Today, many Canadian clinicians employ the Lidcombe Program as their treatment of choice for early stuttering, and the demand for Lidcombe Program Clinician Training Workshops is high. This represents a radical shift in approach to the treatment of stuttering in this country. Why have Canadian clinicians embraced the Lidcombe Program? In this chapter, we discuss this question through evaluation of feedback from an exploratory survey sent to clinicians across the country. Other clinical, cultural, and linguistic issues relevant to treating stuttering within the Canadian context are also explored.

Number of Canadian Clinicians Using the Lidcombe Program

Since the Lidcombe Program was first introduced in Canada in 1997, clinicians have eagerly embraced it. Since the first 4-day Lidcombe Program Clinician Training Workshop in March 1999, more than 150 Canadian clinicians have taken part in workshops, and 100 more clinicians will likely be trained by the end of 2002. It is difficult to estimate how many clinicians are following the Lidcombe Program who have not been trained through workshops. Lidcombe Links for the establishment of follow-up and clinical consultation, mentoring of new clinicians, and group problem solving have been created in six Canadian centers. Clinicians representing 8 of 10 Canadian provinces and 2 of 3 territories (The Northwest Territories and Yukon) have been trained in Lidcombe Program workshops that have taken place across Canada. By 2003 there will be a referral base of Lidcombe Program–trained clinicians representing clinics from Newfoundland in the east to British Columbia in the west.

A questionnaire developed by Rosemary Hayhow at Frenchay Hospital, Bristol, in the United Kingdom, was adapted to explore issues relevant to Canadian clinicians. A group of 225 Canadian clinicians who listed fluency as a specialty were sent a short list of questions. Fifty-six (25%) responded. Of those who responded 83% had heard of the Lidcombe Program through Internet and e-mail correspondence, recent literature, professional newsletters, and conferences. The majority of respondents (55%) had first heard about the Lidcombe Program from colleagues. Based on these results, and on the increasing demand for training and the positive feedback received from those who use the program, it would appear that Canadian clinicians are rapidly choosing the Lidcombe Program as their best practice model for early stuttering treatment.

The feedback we have received from clinicians indicates that the move toward adopting the Lidcombe Program results from a lack of confidence in traditionally accepted treatments for early stuttering. The search for treatments that are effective and the Canadian clinician's enthusiasm for parent involvement in treatment make the Lidcombe Program particularly attractive. Additionally, demand for more efficacious treatment in the public sector, where long-term therapy is not mandated, makes the Lidcombe Program a viable alternative to traditional methods. Armed with appropriate guidelines for early intervention, clinicians who might previously have chosen a less direct approach are discovering that this direct behavioral treatment for young stuttering children can be extremely effective.

Historical Perspectives

In the past decades, our U.S. neighbors have strongly influenced choice of best practice in Canada. Both French and English Canadian clinicians have based treatment on models proposed by clinician writers such as Barry Guitar, Woody Starkweather, Hugo Gregory, and Edward Conture. A challenge to the Francophone clinician is that all the treatment literature and research has been conducted with English-speaking children. Direct comparisons to French-speaking children are not always appropriate, and there are no precedents for issues that might arise in treating children whose native language is other than English.

Treatments of choice historically used to treat early stuttering in Canada can be grouped under two categories: (1) indirect parent counseling or environmental manipulation and (2) direct modification of speech. Although those clinicians who treat stuttering as a specialty would be more likely to use a direct fluency-shaping approach, almost all children who are treated by generalist clinicians receive therapy based on indirect methods. In both the English and French communities, the majority of practitioners are generalist therapists and the number of stuttering children that they see is small. Clinicians who support the wait-and-see approach often advocated by physicians are influenced by treatments that have as their focus the removing or reducing of stressful conditions that are presumed to precipitate stuttering. The accepted rationale for this approach is explained by the Demands and Capacities model of early stuttering (see Chapter 3), which proposes that fluency is at risk when environmental demands for speech and communication exceed the child's cognitive, linguistic, motoric, or social-emotional capacities for maintaining stutter-free speech (Adams, 1990; Starkweather & Gottwald, 1990). Procedures designed to reduce communicative pressure, such as those described by Conture (1997), Rustin, Botterill, and Kelman (1996), and Starkweather, Gottwald, and Halfond (1990), would be considered best practice by the majority of clinicians to shape parent–child interactions in preschool children. The focus is solely on parent counseling.

However, group therapy with a small number of children, where the therapist models good rules for communication based on turn taking and not interrupting, also has a place in the Canadian clinic. Parents learn to modify the environment of the child by altering their interactions. For example, parents attempt to slow speech rate, reduce interruptions, and question less. Because of this background, both English and French parents have traditionally been reluctant to directly intervene in the speech of their child.

When choosing direct treatment, Canadian clinicians choose fluency-shaping approaches that offer structured, programmed, criteria-based guidelines such as those proposed by Shine (1988), Costello (1983), and Meyers and Woodford (1992). In addition, the work of Canadians Boberg and Kully (1985) has greatly influenced stuttering treatment. Their fluency-shaping program for adults has been adapted for children.

Inexperienced clinicians tell us that they often rely on commercially available programs for direct treatment. These "kits" provide step-by-step guides to direct therapy, with worksheets, materials, and record-keeping forms included (e.g., Cooper & Cooper, 1985; Meyers & Woodford, 1992; Ryan, 1974; Shine, 1988). Clinicians also frequently follow modified intensive programs such as those offered at the Institute for Stuttering Treatment and Research for adults. Here young children might be taught to speak using modified fluency targets, including belly breathing and gentle starts.

The reliance of Canadian clinicians upon programmed guides for treatment of early stuttering may reflect the limited training in and exposure to early stuttering. The Canadian Association for Speech–Language Pathology and Audiology has recently revised its requirements for practical experience in the area of fluency disorders to only 10 clinical hours required for certification. Indeed, many clinicians are reluctant to treat stuttering due to their limited training and the notion that the treatments are ineffective in maintaining fluency outside the clinic.

Number of Canadian Children Treated with the Lidcombe Program

The Lidcombe Program was introduced in Canada in 1997 at the Montreal Fluency Center. Because best practice at the center was already direct, client centered, and family oriented (an eclectic mix of the work of Susan Meyer-Fosnot, Lena Rustin, Edward Conture, and Hugo Gregory), it was an easy transition. Following several on-site consultations with Lidcombe clinicians and researchers, the first group of 30 Canadian clinicians was trained in a 3-day workshop presented by Elisabeth Harrison. The enthusiastic response from Canadian clinicians resulted in a demand for more training workshops. The first Lidcombe Program Clinician Training Workshop entirely run by Canadian clinicians took place in November 2000.

At the time of writing, 75 children have completed treatment since the Lidcombe Program was introduced at the Montreal Fluency Center. This number includes both preschool-age and school-age children. Approximately 30 of the 75 children are preschool age, have met the speech criteria established for the Lidcombe Program, and are being followed in Stage 2. In the five clinics that currently form the Lidcombe Link, the Lidcombe Program represents best practice. Another 50 children are being followed in those clinics. In the Quebec sample, 80% of the children treated spoke a second language by age 4 years. At least 15 children speaking French as their mother tongue have received the Lidcombe Program in French to date.

A second, smaller group represents those children for whom the Lidcombe Program was not completed. Some of the reasons for not completing the program are related to very young age, lack of parental compliance, poor attendance due to living far from the clinic, or leaving the program before achieving Stage 2.

Clinical Issues in the Canadian Context

As more clinicians are using the Lidcombe Program in clinical practice, those of us involved in mentoring are called upon to assist in problem solving around various clinical issues. Some of these clinical issues are also faced by clinicians in other countries and reflect common problems that arise when working with early stuttering (e.g., how to manage a particularly talkative child or how to adjust treatment to overcome a period of limited progress). However, a number of clinical issues are particularly Canadian in nature. These Canadian issues relate to the nature of Canadian demographics as well as to service delivery models.

Canada is the world's second largest country, spreading over almost 10 million square kilometers. The country is divided into 10 provinces and 3 territories, with a relatively small population approaching 31 million people. Most residents live in urban centers, the majority located in the southern part of the country, close to the U.S. border. For those Canadians who live in rural or remote areas, access to speech–language pathology services can be problematic. Remote regions often have difficulty recruiting clinicians, and those who are recruited tend to work in sole charge positions, covering vast areas and managing large caseloads. Some areas simply do not have access to speech–language pathology services. Thus, one issue facing Canadian clinicians is the challenge of developing distance therapy to meet the needs of remote communities. A few clinicians have attempted to train parents to carry out the Lidcombe Program from a distance using the Internet, phone contact, telehealth, closed circuit television, and exchange of videotapes back and forth. The experiences of these clinicians and those from other countries who have attempted the Lidcombe Program using distance therapy (e.g., Harrison, Wilson, & Onslow, 1999) will need to be examined to determine how to best proceed with distance cases. Distance therapy is still in its infancy in Canada.

To date, most Lidcombe Program treatment in Canada has been carried out in urban centers. Satisfaction with the Lidcombe Program among Canadian clinicians trained in the program is very high. Of 250 clinicians who have attended training workshops, 140 were surveyed prior to the time of writing, and 26 (19%) returned completed questionnaires. In all, 90% of respondents said they "strongly agreed" or "agreed" with the statement that they are satisfied with the program. One respondent marked "don't know" in response to this item, and only one clinician disagreed with it. Seventy-three percent of clinicians indicated that they "agreed" or "strongly agreed" that the Lidcombe Program is effective for eliminating stuttering, whereas 23% marked "don't know." No clinicians indicated disagreement regarding efficacy of the Lidcombe Program. In addition, 85% of respondents indicated that they "agreed" or "strongly agreed" that the Lidcombe Program is well structured and adapted to the client. Some concerns were expressed regarding difficulty of parental implementation. One third of respondents indicated that they "agreed" that the Lidcombe Program is difficult for parents; however, 58% "disagreed" or "strongly disagreed" with that opinion. Also, although the majority felt that children reach Stage 2 quickly (61%), 30% were uncertain. This finding could reflect the inexperience of newly trained clinicians.

Canadian clinicians seem to appreciate the structure of the Lidcombe Program: the involvement of parents in the treatment; the built-in generalization through verbal contingencies in everyday conversations; and the ease of collecting speech measures that are used to conduct the program and to determine the outcome. The frequent, systematic measurement of a stuttering child's speech both within and beyond the clinic represents a significant change for most Canadian clinicians. When clinicians who were not trained to use the Lidcombe Program were asked how they assess treatment outcome, a variety of answers were given. Although most respondents (58%) indicated that they use some objective measure, such as percentage of syllables stuttered or stuttered words per minute, very few mentioned the use of specific criteria to define acceptable outcomes. Type of dysfluency and secondary behaviors were also cited as measures of treatment outcome. Beyond-clinic measures were rarely indicated ("absence of stuttering on homework tapes" was the only mention of anything approaching a beyond-clinic measure). In addition, 35% of clinicians not using the Lidcombe Program wrote that they assess outcome based on children's feelings about their speech and parental perceptions of their children's speech.

Measuring outcomes to determine clinical efficacy is increasingly important in the Canadian context. Publicly funded institutions that treat childhood speech–language disorders, such as hospitals and school boards, frequently have to defend their services against budget cuts. Efficacy data are a powerful defense: An evidence-based intervention is more difficult to eliminate. Furthermore, the quite few treatment sessions required to reach Stage 2 using the Lidcombe Program (Jones, Onslow, Harrison, & Packman, 2000) provides a defense against budget cuts. In the Lidcombe Program, the clinician collects outcome and duration of treatment data in a cost-effective way as part of the therapy, to be used if called upon to defend stuttering treatment services.

Although there are increasing numbers of clinicians in private practice in Canada, most treatment for childhood speech–language disorders takes place in the public sector. There are differences in the funding formulas and eligibility criteria employed by each province in Canada. Therefore, who can access services, where those services will be accessed, and how long the waiting list is varies depending on place of residence. For example, in the provinces of Ontario and Quebec, where 62% of Canadians reside, children up to age 5 years can be seen in hospital settings. Children older than 5 years are eligible for school-based services. In Quebec, the school board clinicians are, by necessity, generalists; they see all children who present with speech and language disorders. They usually have large caseloads and need to prioritize caseloads based on need. A number of school board clinicians in Quebec have expressed privately that stuttering is a low priority compared with more severe communication deficits. In Ontario, school-based services are provided by school boards and by the School Services Program (SSP), funded by the Ministry of Health. School board clinicians generally do all assessments and then consult with teachers and families but do very little direct therapy. The SSP clinicians theoretically do no assessment but provide intervention for stuttering, voice problems, and moderate to severe phonological disorders.

The service delivery models described are cited as responsible for some of the difficulties that Canadian clinicians may experience when attempting to implement the Lidcombe Program in the public sector. For example, if a child begins the Lidcombe Program at a hospital but has his 5th birthday part way through the treatment, technically that child is no longer eligible to be seen in that setting. The child should be transferred to receive school-based services. Although the transition and the change of therapist are not necessarily detrimental to treatment, most school clinicians have not been trained in the Lidcombe Program. Thus, the Lidcombe Program would either be discontinued or replaced by another treatment by a clinician who has not benefited from Lidcombe Program training. Similarly, if a child turns 5 years old during Stage 2, the school clinician would then complete that stage of treatment. Apart from the issue of whether the school clinician has received Lidcombe Program training, there is the issue of the rapport developed between the original clinician, child, and parents, as well as familiarity with the family and thus with possible problems that could arise during Stage 2. A clinician less familiar with the family will likely have more difficulty problem solving during Stage 2 of the Lidcombe Program.

Another issue that arises from the treatment of children in hospital and school settings is related to the service delivery model employed. Because of the demand for treatment, clinicians are encouraged to see children in groups, to provide treatment in blocks of time, or to treat semimonthly. As the Lidcombe Program is individualized for each child and family, group treatment would likely be problematic. Also, to date, the efficacy of using groups to provide portions of the Lidcombe Program—for example, training parents in measurement—has not been evaluated, so the outcome is unknown. Similarly, the effect on treatment outcome of seeing families every 2 weeks, instead of weekly, has not been studied. Finally, many hospital speech pathology departments and school-based services employ a system whereby children are seen weekly for a block of treatment time, such as for 8 weeks, then put "off-block" for the same period. This block system is inconsistent with the Lidcombe Program service delivery model.

Fortunately, a number of clinics in Ontario have bent the rules, at least temporarily, so that stuttering children being treated with the Lidcombe Program can complete treatment. In addition, these children can often continue to be followed past their 5th birthday in the hospital setting. Apparently, an exception was made for the Lidcombe Program in these settings in large part due to evidence from the research literature supporting the program's efficacy and short median treatment time.

Another issue that frequently arises is how to treat stuttering within the context of coexisting speech and language problems (see Chapter 10). In the public system, there is no structure for referral of children with concomitant speech–language problems for the nonstuttering part of their intervention. If a child stutters and presents with a concomitant language or phonological disorder, the same clinician usually has to address these treatment issues. Clinicians frequently ask if phonological or language goals can be combined with the Lidcombe Program so that two disorders can be treated simultaneously. Or, if two communication disorders are to be treated consecutively, not simultaneously, clinicians ask which disorder should be addressed first. These questions are often debated in clinical problem-solving days. However, to date, there is no published research dealing with the combination of the Lidcombe Program with speech–language interventions. Each case, therefore, needs to be evaluated individually. For example, if stuttering is to be treated first, therapy for the other disorder is recommended when the child reaches maintenance for fluency. If the child's stutter has improved but further progress appears to be hindered by the concomitant disorder, it might be suggested that parents try to maintain the child's fluency at the current level while spending some time on language or phonological goals. A return to stuttering treatment would then occur when those language or phonological goals are met. When a highly unintelligible child is younger than 4 years of age, doing the Lidcombe Program after phonological interventions might be warranted.

We have discussed with clinicians the challenges associated with conducting the Lidcombe Program in a school setting. School-based clinicians have reported that parent attendance can be a problem. Unlike hospitals or private clinics, parents do not need to bring their child to the school treatment setting. Because the Lidcombe Program cannot be done without the parents, school-based clinicians have had to use creative negotiation with parents to arrange meeting times and to thoroughly explain the rationale behind parental involvement. One clinician surveyed wrote that she relies on phone contact with a parent who cannot always meet at the school.

To investigate further the issue of parent compliance, Lidcombe Program–trained clinicians were asked to rate parent compliance on a scale from 1 to 5 (1 = *very good compliance* and 5 = *poor compliance*). No clinicians rated compliance as "poor." However, 14% of clinicians rated compliance as "below average" (a rating of 4) and 50% of clinicians rated compliance as "average" (a rating of 3). Thirty-six percent of clinicians evaluated parent compliance as "good" to "very good" (ratings of 1 and 2). Specific problems with parental compliance reported by clinicians include neglecting to collect speech measures and resistance to carrying out certain aspects of the treatment. Some clinicians have mentioned that for busy families, in particular when both parents work and the child spends much time at day care, parents report it difficult to find time to do the treatment and to collect speech measures. Problem solving with parents is required to determine how they can work around their schedules to provide treatment for their child. These concerns regarding parent compliance likely represent the difficulty of clinicians making the shift to a parent-based training model.

Of the experienced Lidcombe Program clinicians surveyed, 58% felt that the Lidcombe Program was not difficult for parents to learn. They reported that parents have little difficulty learning to acknowledge and praise stutter-free speech. Of the clinicians surveyed, 57% felt that reinforcing stutter-free speech is "relatively easy" for parents (3 on a scale from 1 to 5); 36% felt that this task is "easy" (a rating of 4); and 7% felt that it is "very easy" (a rating of 5). Similarly, 79% of clinicians rated identification of unambiguous stutters as "easy" or "very easy" for parents. A minority, 14% of respondents, felt that identification of unambiguous stutters is "relatively difficult" for parents (a rating of 2).

Cultural Issues in the Canadian Context

Canada is a multilingual, multicultural society with two official languages (English and French) and a number of nonofficial languages. According to the most recent census data from Statistics Canada (1996), approximately 58% of Canadians speak English as their mother tongue and 24% speak French. The nonofficial languages, in order of number of speakers, include Chinese, Italian, German, Polish, Spanish, Portuguese, Punjabi, Ukrainian, Arabic, Dutch, Tagalog, Greek, Vietnamese, Cree, Inuktitut, and others. Each linguistic group in Canada has its own unique mix of cultural customs, traditions, values, and beliefs that affect how individual families react to stuttering and to stuttering intervention. Frequently, the clinician and the client's family are from different ethnic or cultural backgrounds.

A survey conducted by Crago (1990) examined the extent to which clinicians felt themselves able to provide adequate speech and language services to clients representing minority cultures. Results indicated that more than 80% of clinicians in Canada and the United States rated their training with these populations to be inadequate. In our survey, Canadian clinicians attributed lack of success in stuttering treatment for clients from minority cultures to reduced family involvement, inadequate comprehension of the treatment by the client and family, and lack of parent compliance. Modifications often have to be made in treatment to accommodate the family whose first language is not English. For instance, if the client's and family's competence in the language of the clinician is poor, a translator may be warranted.

Cultural sensitivity is important when working with families whose children have any form of communication disorder. Some considerations include each family's perception of help seeking, their communication style (including rules governing politeness), and the interaction styles between adults and children in the family. Issues that are particularly relevant when providing the Lidcombe Program include family perceptions of health and healing and attitudes toward communication problems. For example, in Ontario there is a large community of recent immigrants from Somalia, and a number of clinicians have expressed dismay when working with some of these Somali families due to cultural and religious factors that shape perceptions of stuttering. Specifically, some Somalis believe that God made their child a particular way and it is inappropriate to intervene to try to alter the child's stuttering. However, there are probably more intracultural than intercultural differences in attitude, so generalizations can be as dangerous as cultural insensitivity (Watson & Kayser, 1994; Wayman, Lynch, & Hanson, 1990).

In general, Canadian clinicians believe that the Lidcombe Program is compatible with Canadian parenting styles. Indeed, 79% of clinicians surveyed indicated that the Lidcombe Program was "very compatible" or "compatible" (ratings of 1 and 2 on a scale from 1 to 5). Only 21% of respondents indicated some concerns about compatibility (ratings of 3 and 4). No clinicians felt that the Lidcombe Program is "not at all compatible" with Canadian parenting styles. Discussion with clinicians reveals two main areas of concern. Some parents are uncomfortable discussing their child's stutter while the child is present. This discomfort likely springs from fears that drawing attention to a stutter will make it worse (see Chapter 3). Once myths about stuttering have been laid to rest and the reasons why openness about stuttering is important are discussed, most parents reportedly overcome this initial discomfort. The second area of concern relates to a child-centered or attachment philosophy of parenting that frowns upon correcting children. One parent who espoused this philosophy was happy to praise the child but refused to correct stutters even though the child responded positively to the clinician's request for corrections.

Child-rearing practices and family composition are other factors to consider when working with families from different cultural groups. These issues influence which family member(s) will be trained to administer the Lidcombe Program. In many English and French Canadian families, the mother alone or both the mother and father of the stuttering child are coached in the Lidcombe Program. Occasionally, the father alone is the primary Lidcombe Program provider, as is common in some Arabic-speaking families. Where the client is from and how long the family has lived in Canada both play roles in this and other issues. Native language is another important issue to consider.

General Bilingual and Multilingual Issues

In Canada it is increasingly difficult to find a child older than 4 years who has not been exposed to a second language. Canadian children fall into at least six distinct and different linguistic groups:

1. First language English
2. First language French
3. First language other than English or French
4. Bilingual, which may include English or French plus a second language of the home or two languages that are input with simultaneous exposure
5. Second language added at age 4 years when the child begins preschool in Canada
6. Second language added after age 4 years

Bilingual language acquisition is the result of early, simultaneous, regular, and continued exposure to more than one language from birth. It is a complex process in which children learn their languages not only from parents but also from grandparents, early childhood educators, playmates, and others. Bilingual language acquisition should be differentiated from second language acquisition, which is defined as the process of learning another language after the basics of the first have been acquired. It has been suggested that some young bilingual children who stutter might use linguistic code mixing as a strategy for coping with stuttering (Karniol, 1992). In general, code mixing occurs when children, lacking sufficient vocabulary to express themselves entirely in each language, borrow from the lexicon of the other language within one utterance. In spite of the finding that code mixing is common among bilingual children, Karniol and others (Mattes & Omark, 1984) concluded that, to prevent stuttering, children should not be exposed to a second language until they have acquired good control of their first language. Imposing this recommendation in a culture such as ours, where bilingualism prevails, is impractical, unrealistic, and possibly unnecessary.

The multilingual nature of Canada presents some interesting and challenging problems in the treatment of early stuttering. In using the Lidcombe Program with bilingual or multilingual children, we had to address the following issues: (a) development of a lexicon for the "language of the Lidcombe Program" that would be understood by French and cultural minority parents, (b) provision of treatment when each parent speaks to the child in a different language, and (c) evaluation of treatment outcomes for bilingual and multilingual children.

Treating Stuttering in Children Whose Primary Language Is French

The first issue to be addressed when working with French-speaking children concerned translation of the terminology used in the Lidcombe Program. Canadian clinicians appeared to have no difficulty in translating most procedures of the Lidcombe Program; however, translating praise for stutter-free speech or requests for self-correction was a challenge. Much effort in the early stages of implementing the program in Canada was directed at adapting expressions such as "Good talking," "That was smooth," and "No bumps." In collaboration with parents, we adapted these utterances to reinforce French-speaking children: "Les mots ont bien glissés," "Les mots coulent bien!" "Bravo, les mots ne sont pas restés pris!" After concentrating on praise, we turned our attention to translation of correction: "Le mot a resté pris, peux-tu le réparer?" and "Ooups! Peux-tu faire glisser le mot ______?" We have an ongoing project in which we ask parents to help us develop a lexicon for terms in languages other than English that are used for praise and correction. Once parents understand the concept, it is easy for them to convey the meaning. In addition to French translations, we are finding words for praise and correction in Spanish, Arabic, Italian, Lithuanian, Farsi, and Yiddish. The critical issue may not be the development of the lexicon in other languages, but the consideration of cultural issues related to child rearing and communication among the cultural minority groups in Canada.

When Each Parent Speaks a Different Language

Some interesting questions regarding the delivery of the Lidcombe Program arise when each parent speaks a different mother tongue in a family where the child is bilingual. A possible, and common, scenario is that the mother speaks to the child in her mother tongue (French) and the father speaks in his mother tongue (English); however, the language used to communicate in the home may be typically only French or English. Grandparents may speak a third language and a caregiver may speak a fourth language, often complicating this scenario. One critical element in early bilingual acquisition is the conditions under which the languages are presented to the child. The relationship between the degree to which the various languages are separated or mixed in the input and the child's ultimate bilingual competence has been the subject of much debate (Genesee, 1989).

Although we encourage parents to pursue bilingualism at home, providing that language skills are developing without difficulty, we suggest some guidelines. These include the recommendation that the child not receive code-mixed sentences on input from the parents. An example of this would be starting a sentence in one language and switching to the second for a word or phrase within that sentence. Code mixing used by the child is accepted as part of development of two languages simultaneously, and we have observed that, in instances of early stuttering, children often code mix when they are having difficulty finding a word, in order to increase the complexity of the utterance or in some cases to facilitate fluency (Shenker, Conte, Gingras, Courcy, & Polomeno, 1998). The parent always presents treatment in his or her mother tongue, although the child may respond in either language. Within-clinic measurements taken by the clinician are in either language, depending on the parent who is doing the therapy. Beyond-clinic measurements, when made by both parents, are separated into L1 and L2.

Evaluation of Treatment in Bilingual and Multilingual Children

Many questions have arisen in evaluating the Lidcombe Program with children whose primary language is other than English, who speak more than one language, or who are introduced to a second language during the preschool years. These include the following:

- Is the treatment outcome using the Lidcombe Program with children speaking French or another first language comparable to that obtained with children speaking English as a first language?
- Will treatment take longer with children who speak other than English?
- Will treatment take longer with the Lidcombe Program when children are bilingual or multilingual?
- Are there any significant differences in clinical outcomes when each parent speaks a different language on input?
- Is time to recovery affected when a second language is added when the child is 4 to 5 years of age?

Our preliminary findings suggest that time to recovery in children who speak French as the first language does not differ significantly from those who speak English as the first language. This supports the observation of French clinicians that the Lidcombe Program has the same outcomes when presented in French.

We continue to collect data to support our observations that bilingual language acquisition does not result in an increase in stuttering. This concurs with the findings of Au-Yeung, Howell, Davis, Charles, and Sackin (2001) that there is no difference between monolingual and bilingual speakers in terms of the likelihood of experiencing stuttering in their lives. In their survey of bilingualism and stuttering, Au-Yeung et al. found that acquiring a second language at around 3 years of age might result in a higher chance of stuttering in girls. The authors suggest that learning a second language during a critical period in language development may interfere with language development. We are in a favorable position in Canada to evaluate this finding as we continue to develop the Lidcombe Program for bilingual and multilingual children.

Conclusion

Canadian clinicians interested in using the Lidcombe Program to treat early stuttering are encouraged to attend a 4-day Lidcombe Program training workshop that includes a follow-up day some 6 months later. The follow-up day gives clinicians an opportunity to present a

Lidcombe Program case and participate in group problem solving if needed. Clinicians using the Lidcombe Program are encouraged to remain in contact with, and seek assistance by e-mail or telephone from, the workshop trainers. They may also attend any scheduled follow-up day. In some areas, regular meetings have been set up for clinicians who would like to do more group problem solving than can be provided by a single follow-up day. In spite of the various ways newly trained Canadian clinicians can obtain assistance, the growing number of trained clinicians creates new challenges in managing the Lidcombe Program as best practice across provinces, languages, clinical settings, and clinicians.

We believe that mentoring is required to become competent with the Lidcombe Program; unfortunately, however, not all clinicians who run into difficulty ask for help. Also, at present, only a few clinicians are in a position to mentor colleagues. However, as more clinicians become competent in carrying out the Lidcombe Program, they too will become clinical mentors. One of the clichés often said of Canada is that, in contrast to the individualistic nature of our American neighbors to the south, Canadians are known for their cooperative spirit. That spirit of cooperation will be essential to the success of the Lidcombe Program as the best practice model for treatment of early stuttering in Canada.

References

Adams, M. (1990). The demands and capacities model: I. Theoretical elaboration. *Journal of Fluency Disorders, 15,* 135–141.

Au-Yeung, J., Howell, P., Davis, S., Charles, N., & Sackin, S. (2001). *University College London survey of bilingualism and stuttering.* Unpublished manuscript.

Boberg, E., & Kully, D. (1985). *Comprehensive stuttering treatment program.* San Diego: College-Hill Press.

Conture, E. (1997). Evaluating childhood stuttering. In R. F. Curlee & G. M. Siegel (Eds.), *Nature and treatment of stuttering: New directions* (2nd ed., pp. 239–256). Boston: Allyn & Bacon.

Cooper, E., & Cooper, C. (1985). *Personalized fluency control therapy.* Allen, TX: DLM.

Costello, J. M. (1983). Current behavioral treatments for children. In D. Prins & R. J. Ingham (Eds.), *Treatment of stuttering in early childhood: Methods and issues* (pp. 60–11). San Diego: College-Hill Press.

Crago, M. (1990). Professional gatekeeping: The multicultural, multilingual challenge. *Communique, 4*(1), 10–13.

Genesee, F. (1989). Early bilingual development: One language or two? *Journal of Child Language, 16,* 161–179.

Harrison, E., Wilson, L., & Onslow, M. (1999). Distance intervention for early stuttering with the Lidcombe Programme. *Advances in Speech–Language Pathology, 1,* 31–36.

Jones, M., Onslow, M., Harrison, E., & Packman, A. (2000). Treating stuttering in young children: Predicting treatment time in the Lidcombe Program. *Journal of Speech, Language, and Hearing Research, 43,* 1440–1450.

Karniol, R. (1992). Stuttering out of bilingualism. *First Language, 12,* 255–283.

Mattes, L. J., & Omark, D. R. (1984). *Speech and language assessment for bilingual handicap.* San Diego: College-Hill Press.

Meyers, S. M., & Woodford, L. L. (1992). *The fluency development system for young children.* Buffalo, NY: United Educational Services.

Rustin, L., Botterill, W., & Kelman, E. (1996). *Assessment and therapy for young dysfluent children.* London: Whurr Publishers.

Ryan, B. (1974). *Programmed therapy for stuttering in children and adults.* Springfield, IL: Thomas.

Shenker, R. C., Conte, A., Gingras, A., Courcy, A., & Polomeno, L. (1998). The impact of bilingualism on developing fluency in the preschool child. In E. C. Healey & H. F. M. Peters (Eds.), *Proceedings of the 2nd World Congress on Fluency Disorders* (pp. 200–204). Nijmegen, The Netherlands: Nijmegen University Press.

Shine, R. E. (1988). *Systematic fluency training for young children* (3rd ed.). Austin, TX: PRO-ED.

Starkweather, C. W., & Gottwald, S. (1990). The demands and capacities model: II. Clinical applications. *Journal of Fluency Disorders, 15,* 143–157.

Starkweather, C. W., Gottwald, S., & Halfond, M. (1990). *Stuttering prevention: A clinical method*. Englewood Cliffs, NJ: Prentice Hall.

Statistics Canada. (1996). Population by mother tongue, 1996 census. Retrieved April 12, 2002, from http://www.statcan.ca/english/Pgdb/People/Population/demo18a.htm

Watson, J. B., & Kayser, H. (1994). Assessment of bilingual/bicultural children and adults who stutter. *Seminars in Speech and Language*, *15*, 149–164.

Wayman, K. I., Lynch, E. W., & Hanson, M. J. (1990). Home-based early childhood services: Cultural sensitivity in a family systems approach. *Topics in Early Childhood Special Education*, *10*, 65–66.

Chapter 14

New Zealand

Mark Jones, Marjorie Blakeley, and Tika Ormond

This chapter outlines the stuttering treatments used in New Zealand from the 1940s to the present time. The main focus is the introduction of the Lidcombe Program into New Zealand in the late 1990s. A randomized controlled trial to evaluate the effectiveness of the Lidcombe Program is currently under way in Christchurch and Auckland. The rationale and design of this trial are discussed and progress so far is presented. Results of a survey of New Zealand speech therapists, undertaken in 2001, are also presented. This survey collected information on the treatments currently used by New Zealand speech therapists and on clinical and cultural issues in the New Zealand context.

Historical Perspectives

Documentation of early treatment practices during the 1940s came from the speech therapy training school in Christchurch (Saunders, 1946). This document indicated that treatment should be general, adults should take no notice of the child's stutter, and their manner must suggest "reassurance, patience and gentleness; calmness and stability" (p. 14). Emphasis was placed on personal adjustment by the child to his or her environment, and it was important that stress be eliminated until the child feels that he or she can deal with the situation. Saunders suggested that the child should be given praise for acceptable behavior, and that "every endeavour must be made to supply the child with daily doses of success and achievement, adventure and happiness, rest and relaxation, appreciation, friendship and adequate love!" (p. 14).

In the 1950s a senior therapist on the staff of the Speech Clinic, Cranmer Square, Christchurch, presented a paper to the Conference of New Zealand Speech Therapists (Stroobant, 1952). Stroobant took a sample of 30 stuttering children from the Christchurch Speech Clinic and undertook a psychological investigation to review some of the possible implications for practical and clinical work with children exhibiting stuttering. The results suggested that the sort of therapeutic measures likely to be most effective would require careful choice. In planning a program for each individual, five aspects of treatment were suggested for particular emphasis:

1. Identification of neurotic cases
2. The relearning and practice of fluent patterns of speaking
3. Relief from embarrassment, self-consciousness, and tension
4. Improved adaptability to social relationships
5. Environmental changes

Also in the 1950s a senior member of the Christchurch Speech Clinic staff conducted a controlled experimental study on therapy for her master's thesis (Densem, 1955). Two groups of 10 children were matched with respect to age, gender, and intelligence. The age range of the control group was 6 years 9 months to 13 years 10 months, with a mean of 10 years 5 months, and the range of the experimental group was 6 years 4 months to 13 years 10 months, with a mean of 10 years 5 months. Both groups were treated for stuttering over a 9-week period, attending four times weekly for half-hour sessions. The average attendance was 32.3 sessions for the control group and 31.7 sessions for the experimental group.

Three speech therapists rated the severity of each child's stuttering at the beginning and end of treatment using a 5-point scale. They also judged whether the child had made much improvement, some improvement, or no change. The control group received treatment according to the method generally used in speech clinics in New Zealand, which was based on a statement of the method of treating stuttering supplied by the staff of the Christchurch Speech Clinic. The experimental group received, in addition, direct retraining of the stuttering behavior according to an interpretation based on a reinforcement theory of learning (Sheehan, 1951).

The results from this study suggested that half the children in each group had improved during the 9-week period; hence the additional treatment administered to the experimental children appeared to have no additional benefit. Results suggested, however, that different treatments suit different children; for example, correction should not be used for aggressive or negative children. Also, Densem concluded that positive feeling toward the therapist seems to be necessary before the child will accept guidance in learning.

It seems that psychologists also had opinions on the treatment of early stuttering in the 1950s. Jeffery (1959), a senior psychologist at the Psychological Service, Education Department, Auckland, suggested that stuttering therapy should include

- Building the child's self-confidence
- Ignoring unnecessary mannerisms that the child may have adopted to get his speech under way
- Making the treatment sessions approximate real-life situations
- Encouragement of the child to talk as much as possible
- Introduction of a stable routine of living and not drawing attention to the child's disability

The 1960s saw the advent of group therapy as a possible improvement on individual treatment for stuttering in young children. Nancy Caughley, the lecturer in charge of speech therapy training at the Teachers College in Christchurch, shared her first experience with group therapy in an article (Caughley, 1961). Caughley used two groups of children to trial group therapy for the treatment of stuttering; one group comprised 7 younger children ages 7 to 11 years, and the other group comprised 10 older children ages 10 to 14 years. The treatment included relaxation; discussion of problems with speech; and activities such as mime, charades, and spoken drama. The younger children also were involved with puppetry. Other activities that proved useful and popular were singing and rhythmic choral speaking, quizzes of all kinds, short prepared talks, impromptu speeches, group games involving speech role-playing, and acting out everyday situations. Both groups also practiced such things as telephoning, delivering messages, shopping, and ordering meals in a restaurant.

Providing the groups were carefully chosen and homogeneous with respect to intelligence and social maturity, Caughley (1961) considered that group therapy had advantages over individual therapy, such as the more natural speech situation, the possibility of more interesting activities, the feeling of having a common problem, the stimulus of friendly competition, the possible elimination of self-consciousness, and the minimization of the possibility of the child's becoming overdependent on the therapist. There were also disadvantages, such as the child not being able to talk as freely in a group environment; speech defects being highly individual, thus requiring individual treatment; and some children becoming distressed by seeing their disability in others. Children with these characteristics are best treated individually.

In the 1970s Van Riper's (1973) techniques were used. Workshops on these techniques were given throughout the country by Joan George, a Canadian therapist. Therapists worked conscientiously on "pullouts" and "cancellations" and the approach appeared to be effective, but now only anecdotal evidence is available from worksheets written at the time to support its efficacy. Later, introductions to prolonged speech were carried out at the training school situated at Christchurch College of Education.

The 1980s saw the introduction of treatment based on the work of Rustin, Purser, and Rowley (1987), Goldiamond (1965), Cooper (1971), and Ryan (1979). Clinical researcher Ashley Craig visited New Zealand several times to discuss smooth speech (Goldiamond, 1965) and his work at Prince Henry Hospital in Sydney (Craig, Feyer, & Andrews, 1987). Intensive, smooth speech courses, modeled on those conducted at the Prince Henry Hospital, were run mainly by hospital therapists in the major cities. In the late 1980s the emphasis shifted to direct work with young children as developed by Janis Costello (Costello & Ingham, 1984).

In the 1990s personal construct (Hayhow & Levy, 1987) and prolonged-speech (Onslow & Packman, 1997) techniques were introduced and the Lena Rustin (Rustin et al., 1987) program continued to be used. Mark Onslow visited New Zealand and gave workshops on clinical application of the research with which he was involved with young children who stuttered. From these initial workshops developed a continuing association with the Australian Stuttering Research Centre (ASRC), which has culminated in research being carried out with the ASRC in both the University of Canterbury and the Stuttering Treatment and Research Centre in Auckland. Following establishment of ties with the ASRC, The University of Sydney, and the Stuttering Unit, Bankstown, Sydney, and with two therapists (Marjorie Blakeley and Tika Ormond) completing the training in the Lidcombe Program, there was a dramatic change in service delivery on the University of Canterbury campus. The change has affected not only the early stuttering therapy but also the treatment of advanced stuttering.

Introduction of the Lidcombe Program in New Zealand

The course in clinical management of stuttering has been conducted at the University of Canterbury since 1998. The course was designed by Mark Onslow from the ASRC, and course instructors, Sally Stocker, Anna Huber, and Linda Wilson. This course is presented in an intensive format and is conducted over 1 week. It is designed to be supplemented by clinical practice, made possible by the fact that the Lidcombe Program is being demonstrated in the campus clinics alongside the ongoing Lidcombe Program research program.

The emphasis in this course is on independent learning leading to problem solving, training in the ability to accurately measure stuttering, and developing an understanding of how professional literature informs clinical practice. The students move from lectures to discussion groups with a high expectation of participation and group and individual problem solving. Students involved in the course have consistently given positive reviews on their learning and from reports would appear to be using the Lidcombe Program as graduates in their work setting.

At the time of writing, the Department of Speech and Language Therapy at the University of Canterbury is the only venue in New Zealand for training speech–language therapists, so courses presented at that university have a major impact on treatment in New Zealand. The Stuttering Treatment and Research Trust in Auckland is also involved in a research project on the Lidcombe Program, which is presently being conducted by a graduate who attended the course in clinical management of stuttering at Canterbury.

A Randomized Controlled Trial of the Lidcombe Program

Introduction

In mid-1998 discussion began between the ASRC and the University of Canterbury about the possibility of a research project in New Zealand to evaluate the effectiveness of the Lidcombe Program. The Lidcombe Program was fairly well entrenched in a large part of Australia, whereas it was quite novel in New Zealand. In fact, it seemed there was no formal treatment offered to preschool-age children in New Zealand. It was thought this would provide an ideal opportunity to do a large-scale clinical trial to establish the effectiveness of the Lidcombe Program for treating early stuttering.

The research project was planned to be a collaboration between the University of Canterbury and the ASRC. The University of Canterbury would provide the treatment for the children, and the ASRC would oversee the project. After a protocol for the trial was written and approved by the ethics committees from the University of Canterbury and The University of Sydney, a randomized controlled trial (RCT) commenced, with the first children randomized in June 1999. A brief outline of the project follows (see Jones, Gebski, Onslow, & Packman, 2000).

Background

At the time the RCT commenced, a number of studies had already shown favorable outcomes for the Lidcombe Program (Lincoln & Onslow, 1997; Lincoln, Onslow, & Reed, 1997; Onslow, Andrews, & Lincoln, 1994; Onslow, Costa, & Rue, 1990). Jones, Onslow, Harrison, and Packman (2000) showed that children age 2 through 6 years can have Lidcombe Program treatment delayed for at least 1 year post-onset without compromising the time taken for successful treatment. This is important information in the development of the RCT of the Lidcombe Program because it is possible that control children in that trial will not receive any treatment for 9 months (as discussed later).

For decades it had been thought that stuttering is caused by environmental influences that make speech troublesome for children. Not surprisingly, then, concerns have been raised that Lidcombe Program methods might have an adverse psychological impact on children because the treatment is conducted by parents and because it involves drawing the child's attention to stuttering (Cook, 1996; Cook & Rustin, 1997). Hence an important part of the development of the RCT has been an investigation of its safety in terms of psychological impact on children. Woods, Shearsby, Onslow, and Burnham (2002) assessed children before and after the treatment for signs of anxiety, aggression, withdrawal, or depression, and for signs of deterioration in the quality of attachment between mother and child. There were no signs of any such changes, and in fact data suggested that the procedure resulted in a positive psychological impact.

In sum, the collective weight of evidence from these preliminary studies suggested that the Lidcombe Program was a promising new treatment that warranted a large-scale trial. To date, all children reported in outcome studies have attained and maintained near-zero stuttering for clinically significant periods, and social validity and safety investigations have been positive. Consequently, a large-scale RCT of the Lidcombe Program has commenced in New Zealand.

At the time the RCT began, the Lidcombe Program was not considered standard practice for early stuttering in New Zealand and it was not routinely presented to children who began to stutter. The Christchurch area is the preliminary point of contact for the study. Preliminary investigations determined that, at the time the study began, there was no generally accepted treatment for stuttering preschool children in that area, with some clinicians using variants of Goldiamond's (1965) prolonged-speech procedure adapted for children, and family counseling based on Rustin's procedures (Rustin, Botterill, & Kelman, 1996). However, at the time the trial started, the majority of preschool children in the Christchurch area were not treated. Hence the standard practice control group for the RCT is, generally, no formal treatment, with some cases being treated as outlined above. Reasons for considering no formal treatment to be the best practice include an absence of direct evidence to the contrary, and a belief that children are best treated when they are more mature and unlikely to recover naturally.

The RCT, therefore, is a pragmatic trial, addressing the following fundamental question: Is treatment with the Lidcombe Program superior to current standard practice? The control treatment is what would normally be given to children if the Lidcombe Program were not available. Under these conditions, it is admissible to have more than one method of treatment in the control arm of the trial.

Hypotheses

The primary hypothesis is that 9 months after beginning treatment, %SS will be lower by at least 1 percentage point for those children undergoing the Lidcombe Program. In addition, it is likely that a number of the control children will spontaneously recover, so the time taken to achieve less than 1%SS will be evaluated. It is hypothesized that the children treated with the Lidcombe Program will have shorter times to achieve less than 1%SS.

Subject Selection

Eligibility Criteria

A child must meet the following criteria to participate in the study:

- Age at enrollment must be from 3 to 6 years, inclusive.
- The child must be diagnosed as stuttering using standard procedures.
- The child and parents must be proficient in English.

Pretreatment assessment, confirmation of eligibility, and obtaining of informed consent is completed for each child prior to inclusion into the study.

Exclusion Criteria

A child who meets any of the following criteria is excluded from the study:

- Severity of stuttering is less than 2%SS.
- The child has been treated in the previous 12 months for stuttering.
- The onset of stuttering was less than 6 months prior to date of randomization.

Randomization Procedures

Children are randomly allocated either to the Lidcombe Program or to standard practice treatment. Factors that possibly influence treatment success can be taken account of in the randomization process by stratification. Stratification ensures that approximately equal numbers of subjects are allocated to each treatment within important subgroups (strata). Stratification factors (with strata specified in brackets) for this study are as follows:

- Rate of stuttering (<5%SS vs. >5%SS)
- Age at enrollment (<4 years vs. >4 years)
- Family history of recovery where at least one first-degree relative has recovered from stuttering (yes vs. no)
- Gender (male vs. female)

Treatment Plans

The children in the Lidcombe Program group receive the program as set out in the treatment manual (Australian Stuttering Research Centre, 2002). In the standard practice group, each child and at least one parent have an initial consultation with the clinician where the trial is explained and baseline speech measures and demographic characteristics are collected. After the initial consultation, the parent provides recordings of the child's speech at the times outlined in the following section and documents any treatment for stuttering given to the child.

Study Parameters and Assessments

Timing of Assessments

For the purposes of measuring outcome, all children in both groups are audiorecorded by their parents using domestic tape recorders in three beyond-clinic speaking situations: speaking to a family member at home, speaking to a nonfamily member at home, and speaking to a nonfamily member away from home. Parents present a tape containing the three recordings at each assessment occasion. Pretreatment assessments occur 2 weeks and 1 week prior to randomization. Postrandomization assessments occur over a 9-month period: at 1 week, 1 month, 2 months, 3 months, 4 months, 6 months, and 9 months.

Speech Measures

The speech recordings are assessed by an experienced clinician for %SS. These measures are made on samples of speech of at least 300 syllables and involve the use of an electronic button-press counter/timer. The clinicians are blinded to the identity of the child and the group to which the child belongs.

Statistical Considerations

To achieve a power of 80%, with a significance level of .05, based on the primary outcome, a sample size of 55 is required in each treatment arm. This calculation allows a drop-in rate and drop-out rate of 10%; in other words, up to 10% of children can drop out of the Lidcombe Program and up to 10% of the control children can be treated with the Lidcombe Program.

Progress

At the time of writing, the trial had recruited 38 children in total, 25 from Christchurch and 13 from Auckland. A number of issues have arisen throughout the progress of the trial, the main two being rate of recruitment and control group delinquency. It was hoped that 1 child could be recruited to the study per week but it turns out that 1 child per month is more realistic. Also, obtaining speech tapes for the control group children is proving difficult. The recruitment from Christchurch is slow as it seems that word has spread that the Lidcombe Program appears to work very well and parents can receive the Lidcombe Program for their children from other sources. In an effort to increase recruitment, the Stuttering Treatment and Research Trust in Auckland joined the trial in 2001. Other sites may join the trial sometime in the future.

Survey of New Zealand Speech–Language Therapists

In early 2001, a questionnaire was sent to speech–language therapists in New Zealand asking questions about the treatment of stuttering. Fifty-nine responses were obtained from a cross-section of speech–language therapists working in schools, hospitals, and independent practice. A summary of the results can be found in Tables 14.1 to 14.3.

The participants were asked to report what treatments they used for children and adults who stutter. The responses are shown in Table 14.1. Nearly all respondents reported they used elements from more than one program depending on the client's individual needs. The following combinations were named:

- Gradual Increase in Length & Complexity of Utterance (GILCU; Ryan, 1974), Smooth Speech (Nielson & Andrews, 1993)
- GILCU, Easy Does It (Heinze & Johnson, 1985), Lidcombe Program
- Lena Rustin (Rustin et al., 1996), Smooth Speech, Lidcombe Program
- Smooth Speech, Prolonged-Speech (Onslow & Packman, 1997), Lena Rustin
- Lena Rustin, Smooth Speech
- Lidcombe Program, Easy Does It
- Lidcombe Program, Smooth Speech
- Easy Does It, Smooth Speech
- Smooth Speech, GILCU

The 59 respondents reported that the number of clients treated for stuttering in the year 2000 ranged from 1 to 23, with an average of 7. This represented an average of less than 7% (range: 0.5% to 17%) of their total workload.

Table 14.2 presents the opinions of the 59 respondents when asked to indicate the clinical issues they deemed important in the delivery of stuttering treatments. *Service delivery* was seen as an important clinical issue because of the large time commitment needed for the intensive nature of follow-up and data analysis. *Matching programs to individual needs* was also important due to the difficulty of working with clients who have a learning disability, speak English as a second language, and stutter. There were also problems with caregiver support and program implementation. Others thought that there was a reliance on the competency level of the therapist by parents and teachers, which raises expectations that the therapist can treat the child without involving other caregivers. Of slightly less importance was *variability of stuttering as a disorder.* Of least importance seemed to be the *recorded differences between researchers' findings*. Some respondents indicated a need for specialist centers for stuttering.

Table 14.1 Treatment Programs Used by 59 Speech–Language Therapists in New Zealand.

Treatment Program	How Many Use It	Range of Clients
Lena Rustin	13	Children
Lidcombe	42	Children
Smooth Speech	47	Adults and children
Naturalness	10	Adults
Easy Does It	19	Children
Personal Construct	8	Adults
Cognitive Behavior Therapy	6	Adults
Gradual Increase in Length & Complexity of Utterance	11	Older school children

Table 14.2 Clinical Issues in the Treatment of Stuttering Deemed Important by 59 Respondents.

Clinical Issues	How Many Agree
Service delivery	48
Matching programs to individual needs	33
Variability of stuttering as a disorder	24
Recorded differences between researchers' findings	8

Table 14.3 Cultural Issues in the Treatment of Stuttering Considered Important by 59 Respondents.

Cultural Issues	How Many Agree
The need for family involvement	47
Family priorities	36
The format of some programs	23

Table 14.3 shows the cultural issues the respondents considered important in the delivery of stuttering treatments. The *need for family involvement* was seen as an important cultural issue with these subissues: the expectation of the expert to fix the problem, the difficulty of motivating school-age children, and the inability of working parents to devote time to the treatment program. The *formats of some programs* do not suit some cultural groups and need to be adapted. *Family priorities* are also important because some families are too busy to provide follow-up. Clinicians need to consider the family's cultural priorities when developing treatment programs. For example, English as a second language can cause difficulty in understanding the program, and sometimes clinicians find it hard to communicate what the family can provide. There is a need for more user-friendly models that can accommodate such things as weekend and evening appointments and a family-based course.

Conclusion

This chapter has traced the history of early stuttering intervention in New Zealand from the 1940s to the introduction of the Lidcombe Program in the late 1990s. Approaches to early intervention have historically been eclectic and at the time of this writing remain so, judging by the results of a recent survey of New Zealand therapists. According to that survey, there is no clear preference for any one treatment for early stuttering in New Zealand, with respondents reporting that they used a variety of interventions and, indeed, frequently combined elements of different approaches. This, then, provides support for not having any one treatment for the control group in the RCT.

References

Australian Stuttering Research Centre. (2002). *Manual for the Lidcombe Program of early stuttering intervention*. Retrieved April 12, 2002, from http://www.fhs.usyd.edu.au/asrc/treatment/lid_manual.htm

Caughley, N. (1961). Group therapy in the speech clinic—The pros and cons. *New Zealand Speech Therapists' Association Journal, 16*, 24–27.

Cook, F. (1996, April). The Lidcombe Programme—Is this the cure? *Bulletin of the Royal College of Speech and Language Therapists, 528*, p. 14.

Cook, F., & Rustin, L. (1997). Commentary on the Lidcombe Program of early stuttering intervention. *European Journal of Disorders of Communication, 32*, 250–258.

Cooper, E. B. (1971). Integrating behaviour therapy and traditional insight treatment procedures with stuttering. *Journal of Communication Disorders, 4*, 40–43.

Costello, J. M., & Ingham, R. J. (1984). Assessment strategies for stuttering. In R. F. Curlee & W. H. Perkins (Eds.), *Nature and treatment of stuttering: New directions* (pp. 303–333). San Diego: College-Hill Press.

Craig, A. R., Feyer, A. M., & Andrews, G. (1987). An overview of a behavioral treatment for stuttering. *Australian Psychologist, 22*, 53–62.

Densem, A. E. (1955). The treatment of stammering (An interpretation according to a reinforcement theory of learning): An outline of some recent research. *New Zealand Speech Therapists' Association Journal, 10*, 3–11.

Goldiamond, I. (1965). Stuttering and fluency as manipulatable operant response classes. In L. Krasner & L. P. Ullman (Eds.), *Research in behavior modification* (pp. 106–156). New York: Holt, Rinehart & Winston.

Hayhow, R., & Levy, C. (1987). *Working with stuttering: A personal construct therapy approach*. Bicester, UK: Winslow Press.

Heinze, B. A., & Johnson, K. L. (1985). *Easy does it: Fluency activities for young children*. East Moline, IL: LinguiSystems.

Jeffery, R. J. (1959). Stammering—A two-dimensional theory. *New Zealand Speech Therapists' Association Journal, 14*, 18–24.

Jones, M., Gebski, V., Onslow, M., & Packman, A. (2000, April). *Rationale, methods, and design of a randomised controlled trial of the Lidcombe Program of early stuttering intervention*. Poster presentation at the Society for Clinical Trials meeting, Toronto.

Jones, M., Onslow, M., Harrison, E., & Packman, A. (2000). Treating stuttering in young children: Predicting treatment time in the Lidcombe Program. *Journal of Speech, Language, and Hearing Research, 43*, 1440–1450.

Lincoln, M., & Onslow, M. (1997). Long-term outcome of an early intervention for stuttering. *American Journal of Speech–Language Pathology, 6*, 51–58.

Lincoln, M., Onslow, M., & Reed, V. (1997). Social validity of an early intervention for stuttering: The Lidcombe Program. *American Journal of Speech–Language Pathology, 6*, 77–84.

Nielson, M., & Andrews, G. (1993). Intensive fluency training of chronic stutterers. In R. F. Curlee (Ed.), *Stuttering and related disorders of fluency* (pp. 139–165). New York: Thieme Medical.

Onslow, M., Andrews, C., & Lincoln, M. (1994). A control/experimental trial of an operant treatment for early stuttering. *Journal of Speech and Hearing Research, 37*, 1244–1259.

Onslow, M., Costa, L., & Rue, S. (1990). Direct early intervention with stuttering: Some preliminary data. *Journal of Speech and Hearing Disorders, 55,* 405–416.

Onslow, M., & Packman, A. (1997). Designing and implementing a strategy to control stuttered speech in adults. In R. F. Curlee & G. M. Siegel (Eds.), *Nature and treatment of stuttering: New directions* (2nd ed., pp. 357–376). Boston: Allyn & Bacon.

Rustin, L., Botterill, W., & Kelman, E. (1996). *Assessment and therapy for young disfluent children.* London: Whurr Publishers.

Rustin, L., Purser, H., & Rowley, D. (1987). *Progress in the treatment of fluency disorders.* London: Taylor & Francis.

Ryan, B. P. (1974). *Programmed therapy for stuttering in children and adults.* Springfield, IL: Thomas.

Ryan, B. P. (1979). Stuttering therapy in a framework of operant conditioning and programmed learning. In H. H. Gregory (Ed.), *Controversies about stuttering therapy* (pp. 129–173). Baltimore: University Park Press.

Saunders, M. E. (1946). Notes on the treatment of stammering. *New Zealand Speech Therapists' Association Journal, 1,* 14–15.

Sheehan, J. (1951). The modification of stuttering through non-reinforcement. *Journal of Abnormal Psychology, 46,* 51–63.

Stroobant, R. E. (1952). A psychological study of some stammering children. *New Zealand Speech Therapists' Journal, 7*(2).

Van Riper, C. (1973). *The treatment of stuttering.* Englewood Cliffs, NJ: Prentice Hall.

Woods, S., Shearsby, J., Onslow, M., & Burnham, D. (2002). Psychological impact of the Lidcombe Program of early stuttering intervention: Eight case studies. *International Journal of Language & Communication Disorders, 37,* 31–40.

Chapter 15

South Africa

Margaret Marks Wahlhaus, Joan Girson, and Caron Levy

Historical Perspectives

From the 1930s onward, theory and treatment of stuttering in South Africa were dominated by the philosophy of the Iowa school (for an overview, see Ingham, 1984 and Chapter 3). This philosophy was brought to our country in the late 1930s by Alan Clemons, who had been one of Wendell Johnson's students. Clemons, who stuttered himself, taught at the University of the Witwatersrand, Johannesburg, which was, at that time, the only South African university that had a course in communication disorders, which at the time was called logopedics.

The reluctance to label a child's stuttering as such constituted the prevailing thinking and practice of the time. This is perhaps not surprising, given that stuttering was considered as diagnosogenic in that it was said to be caused by parental labeling of the child's normally disfluent speech as "stuttering." As Johnson (1955) expressed the essence of his theory, "stuttering . . . would seem to start, not in the speaker's mouth, but in the listener's ear" (p. 11). According to that theory, drawing attention to a child's normal disfluencies created awareness that speech was "wrong." Consequently, the child would try to to hide the "wrong" behavior and would introduce tension and effort into speech; this would have the effect of making normal disfluency into stuttering. What would have been easy repetitions or hesitations would come to be accompanied by struggle behaviors, as the progressive primary and secondary stages of the condition evolved along the lines described by Bluemel (1935). Together with this speech deterioration would come negative feelings about speech and speaking situations. Consequently, it was considered imperative that the child not become aware that there was anything about his or her speech that was aberrant.

This type of thinking barred many clinicians from making a diagnosis of stuttering. It was felt safer to watch and wait. The influence of the diagnosogenic theory meant that there was little, if any, direct work done on early stuttering in South Africa from the 1930s on. If the young child did receive some attention, it was typically indirect therapy that attempted to build up language skills and feelings that speech was pleasant and easy. Some clinicians, particularly those with a psychodynamic leaning, conducted some form of play therapy. The majority of treatment time was spent working alone with parents, advising them on ways of reducing stressors on the child, particularly communication stressors.

It is tempting to assert, with hindsight, that these early therapies were without any benefit. Although not documented in scientific journals, reports of progress and personal experience of clinicians working during those years indicated that many of the young children did improve, often to the point of stopping stuttering altogether. Of course, many of the children may not have really been stuttering but were, as the diagnosogenic theory asserted, passing through a stage of disfluency that was part of the normal development and acquisition of speech and language proficiency. As outcome measurements were not as often used in treatement then as now, it is not possible to evaluate the efficacy of those early treatments in any scientific manner.

As with many academics and practitioners in the Western world, South African workers were faced with conflicting ideas about stuttering. One of the most difficult issues, which still presents controversy, is associated with the fractious questions surrounding the difficulties in defining stuttering (Marks Wahlhaus, 1990). Many of these questions can be viewed as semantic problems, but also have clinical implications. Questions arise such as these: Can we accept the concept of stuttering-like disfluencies (Yairi & Ambrose, 1992), or are these another way of describing stuttering behavior? Should nonspeech parameters be taken into account when a diagnosis is made and consequent intervention program is embarked on? What behaviors must a young child show to merit intervention? Is diagnosis a matter of quantity or quality? These kinds of questions bedeviled those who believed that no direct work could be done with a child unless stuttering was actually diagnosed.

Clearly, however, many clinicians in South Africa had frustrations similar to those outlined by Bloodstein (1986). Clinicians realized that it was difficult to find a child who stuttered and was not aware of it (Levy & Girson, 2001). Also, clinicians queried why, if it was considered acceptable to draw a child's attention to any other communication problem such as misarticulation, stuttering was considered so untouchable that it could not be mentioned without any negative effects. Also, clinicians realized that acknowledgment had to be made of parental pleas that they wanted to do more to help a child struggling with speech than to give an assurance that "I know it is hard for you to talk."

Up to the 1950s the major thinking about psychological issues and problems that affected a person's psychosocial adjustment had been dominated by psychodynamic theorists and practitioners. With these treatments, clients traditionally received long-term analytic treatment based on their individual problems. The use of programs, which were considered as applying a relatively customized approach to clients, was not the usual practice.

In direct contrast, behavior modification based on learning principles had strong advocates such as Wolpe and his associates, who were working in South Africa (Wolpe, 1958). These professionals helped bring about a reorientation of thought about stuttering. There was recognition of the fact that stuttering should be viewed as a behavior that could be treated using the principles of behavior modification. Speech clinicians began to accept that it could be beneficial to use some programs that had been developed along these lines. Acceptance was accorded to the concept of operant conditioning and programmed instruction. Many programs were implemented during past decades, such as Shine's (1980) systematic fluency training, as well as procedures based on the principle of increasing the length and complexity of utterances (Costello, 1984; Ryan, 1979). The work of Gregory and Hill (1980) also influenced treatment during past decades, particularly the modeling of easy relaxed speech used to increase the amount of fluency and the introduction of desensitization procedures to increase the tolerance for those factors that disrupt fluency.

In effect, these approaches introduced South African clinicians to the notion of a systematic approach for young stutterers that emphasized the use of the child's existing fluency. This made clinicians ready and welcoming recipients for the approach developed by the Lidcombe workers.

It is interesting to note that an approach incorporating praise for fluent speech had been considered several decades before in South Africa. Asher Bar, visiting South Africa as a guest lecturer in the early 1970s, mentioned that there was an attempt to use the principle of praise for a young stuttering child's fluent speech. Van Riper (1973, p. 383) described Bar's use of "discreetly reinforcing the fluent speech by occasional approvals or the immediate granting of attention." Bar's approach was met with some criticism from the South African clinicians, their reactions being, in essence, "if the child learns that fluent speech is a good thing to do, the immediate corollary is that stuttering is a bad thing to do."

Introduction of the Lidcombe Program in South Africa

The senior author, who had taught stuttering at the University of the Witwatersrand, Johannesburg, for many years, migrated to Australia in the early 1990s. Having met Mark Onslow and his colleagues, she was enthusiastic about the Lidcombe approach and, on a visit to South Africa, introduced it in lectures to postgraduate students as well as to interested speech pathologists. This approach, diametrically opposed to what many had believed and practiced in South Africa, was generally received with much interest as an innovative and beneficial intervention procedure. There was, however, some expressed astonishment that the young child should be in the room, and even in the conversation, when his or her stuttering (previously more delicately labeled "speech difficulty" or "nonfluency") was being discussed openly.

Because of the great interest in his work and that of his associates, Mark Onslow was invited to South Africa by the University of the Witwatersrand in 1997 for a series of undergraduate and graduate lectures, and his presentations of the Lidcombe Program were enthusiastically received. He also lectured at the other teaching universities in the country, and spoke to the general public through the various media, again engendering much interest. Following his visit, two authors of this chapter, Joan Girson and Caron Levy, attended a 2-week workshop in Sydney in June 1998. This workshop involved immersion in therapy observations, lectures, and discussions with staff members of the Australian Stuttering Research Centre and the Stuttering Unit at Bankstown Health Service, Sydney.

Lectures and Workshops

On their return to South Africa, Girson and Levy introduced the Lidcombe Program through lectures and demonstrations to students at the University of the Witwatersrand, and presented papers at local and national conferences (see Levy & Girson, 2001). In answer to the many requests for practical demonstrations, the Australian Stuttering Research Centre was approached to lend its expertise to conduct a workshop.

The first Lidcombe Program workshop was organized in July 1999, and was conducted by Sue O'Brian, a member of the Lidcombe team, who came from Australia specifically for this. Girson and Levy assisted in the running of this most successful venture and, in July 2000, conducted a workshop themselves for 33 graduate clinicians. In October and November of the same year, they were involved in teaching the program to graduate clinicians and to students at the University of the Witwatersrand; the Lidcombe Program is now being taught at several of the South African universities. Girson and Levy act as consultants when questions are raised about the program. There is a proposal for a regular Lidcombe Program discussion group to be started, which will act as a support system for clinicians.

Questionnaire on Workshops

In March 2001, questionnaires were sent to 58 of the graduates who had attended the various workshops, to assess their effectiveness (Levy & Girson, 2001). There were 12 respondents, the small response rate possibly being due in part to a postal strike and to people being out of the country.

Of the 12 respondents, all felt that the workshops had been beneficial and had changed their original impression of traditional stuttering therapy with very young children. However, at the time the information was gathered, only 4 respondents had used the program. The 8 respondents who had not used the Lidcombe Program reported that they either did not work with children or did not yet feel confident in use of the program. The 4 who had used it had treated a total of 20 patients, with an age range from 2 years 6 months to 6 years 0 months, with the Lidcombe Program. The duration of Stage 1 of the program varied from 2 to 12 months, and the results as stated by the respondents were rated as "satisfactory" to "good."

An overview of the responses showed that respondents considered the advantages of the program to include the reduced number of sessions required compared with traditional methods, increased parental involvement, and empowerment of the family in terms of responsibility in the therapy process. Other advantages reported by the clinicians were that intervention could occur in younger children than with conventional methods, and that the program could be undertaken in many languages.

The disadvantages perceived by the respondents were that parents often did not have sufficient time to devote to the implementation of the Lidcombe Program, and did not always attend regularly. The caregivers often did not understand the underlying concepts of the program and consequently did not always administer it correctly. The clinicians noted that, where the child or family had serious problems in addition to stuttering, stuttering was not a priority for parents and they were not motivated to implement the program.

Only one respondent (who had not actually used the treatment) queried the measurement requirements of the Lidcombe Program. It was of interest that no one else mentioned measurement, as several people at the workshops had appeared intimidated by the measurements required during the Lidcombe Program. It was not possible to know if the respondents were using measurements, were using them and having difficulty with them, or were ignoring this aspect of the treatment altogether. Another matter of concern was that some respondents stated they used the Lidcombe Program as part of an eclectic approach, an issue that is discussed later in this chapter.

Summary of Clinical Experiences with the Lidcombe Program in South Africa

This section describes the clinical experiences of two of the authors (Levy and Girson) in administering the Lidcombe Program to 18 clients since their 1998 visit to Lidcombe and Bankstown. Of the 18 children treated, the mean age of onset of stuttering was 3 years 0 months, and the mean age at initial consultation was 4 years 2 months. The caseload comprised 13 boys and 5 girls, 38% of whom had received some type of stuttering therapy previously, and 72% of whom had a family history of stuttering, primarily on the paternal side of the family. Associated speech, language, behavioral, or emotional problems were evidenced in 38% of the children. Of these children, 88% completed Stage 2, or were in Stage 2 at the time of writing. The mean duration of weekly therapy conducted until the beginning of Stage 2 was 10.5 weeks, which is similar to that in other reports about the Lidcombe Program

(Hayhow, Kingston, & Ledzion, 1998; Jones, Onslow, Harrison, & Packman, 2000). The children with additional problems needed more time than those without.

When considering the implementation of any treatment program for stuttering in South Africa, clinicians must consider several issues inherent in the political, social, and cultural conditions in that country (Levy & Girson, 2001). Possibly one of the most prominent is that there are both First and Third World conditions existing in the country. For the First World minority, the problems of stuttering are no different from those in other Western countries; however, for the majority of the remaining nearly 40 million people, with so many difficulties besetting them, stuttering is not considered high on the priority list as a condition warranting attention or state assistance. Consequently, for many, therapy is seldom available, affordable, or accessible.

Additionally, South Africa is a multicultural and multilingual society, which leads to unique problems in the implementation of any therapy. For historical reasons there are wide schisms between various groups within South African society. People are divided by race, language, class, and educational status. As the country moves toward a united society, clinicians are becoming increasingly aware of the challenges these differences present. At present the majority of clinicians are White, middle class, and educated, with limited personal experience of the specific cultures, languages, and problems of daily life confronting other sections of the population from which the majority of the client base comes. Clinicians require sensitivity to the cultural divides between themselves and the caregivers of the stuttering children. These include expectations of therapy; terminology during treatment; and modes of interaction between children and adults, and between professionals and laypeople. Some of these issues that were noted by the authors to affect the clinical presentation of the Lidcombe Program in South Africa are discussed in the following sections.

Social Differences Between Clients and Clinicians

In the very large proportion of client–clinician interactions, the clinician comes from a different background from that of the child and caregiver, and the differences have been underscored by the previous political regime. Not only race but also variables such as the education and social status of the parent affect the way in which the mother perceives and reacts to the clinician, and vice versa. The Lidcombe Program requires that the clinician and caregiver work together in a relationship of mutual trust. This is impossible if the relationship between the caregiver and clinician is one of fear, subservience, and resentment. Although these problems may occur elsewhere in the world and affect the Lidcombe Program, they are particularly noteworthy in the South African context, where for so many years members of different population groups were in defined roles of political and social dominance and submission.

Parents and Caregivers

Our experience has been that many children have little or no contact with their parents, which can make the selection of a participant in the therapy process a difficult one. Some parents work all day and children are left in child care centers or in the care of an au pair or nanny. The parents often leave early and return late and have no time to attend therapy sessions or to work with their children. Some of these caregivers did not consider administration of the Lidcombe Program part of their duties. Other children stayed with grandparents or other relatives during the week, often seeing their parents infrequently for long periods, and then moving on to the parents or another relative on the weekend. Constraints of time, finances, and transport sometimes made it difficult for the caregiver to accompany the child to weekly visits to the clinician, which is an inherent part of the Lidcombe Program. At times, even though the caregiver did attend clinic sessions and did administer the program effectively, difficulties arose because parents were reluctant to be instructed by employed caregivers in methods of handling the child's speech.

Although many parents in the more affluent sections of the population employ nannies to care for their children, those in the poorer sections of the population are forced to leave their children in the care of neighbors, elderly grandparents, or older siblings. In some sectors of the population, parents, particularly fathers, are seen as remote, disciplinarian figures whose contact with the child is usually formal. All these factors have led to a situation where many South African parents do not know how to react comfortably with their children in the way that the Lidcombe Program requires. The notion of providing supportive, verbal-contingent stimulation during everyday conversations can be a difficult and foreign one for these parents to accept and practice. The clinician often has to teach the parent new ways of reacting to the child. This is particularly germane in the administration of requests for self-correction. Levy and Girson (2001) found that many parents and caregivers tended to overuse requests for self-correction, becoming punitive in so doing. With some children they found it necessary to delete correction from the treatment.

Language

There are 11 official languages in South Africa and several unofficial ones. Many children grow up within a multilingual environment. A child may have a Xhosa-speaking father and a Tswana-speaking mother, attend an English medium school, and have neighbors who speak several of the other languages. Decisions had to be made as to which language should be used in therapy. For practical reasons, the clinician usually conducted the formal therapy sessions in English, whereas the parent worked at home with the child in the language of choice. This could sometimes create problems of its own, as the child might prefer English, whereas the parent might be adamant that the child retain and use the mother tongue. It was also sometimes an issue that the parent used a second language, which presented a clinician–parent barrier for effective instruction.

Isolation from Treatment Services

Regular attendance at the clinic was not always possible, often because of the distances that some clients had to travel. In some cases transport difficulties and financial constraints made it difficult for families to attend. This was a matter for each clinician to handle according to the demands of each family's circumstances. Because the Lidcombe Program needs to be administered with parent(s) and child visiting the clinic each week, decisions needed to be made about whether to enroll a child in the treatment if regular attendance could not be managed.

Not surprisingly, then, a number of families in areas where therapy was not available requested that the Lidcombe Program be conducted by distance intervention (Harrison, Wilson, & Onslow, 1999). Some of these requests came from countries beyond the South African borders. Two cases were treated in this way; one had good results but the other was unsuccessful due to adverse family dynamics and the need to refer the child to a local psychotherapist. To conduct distance treatment successfully, both clinician and parent need access to technological support, such as tape recorders, telephones, e-mail, and faxes. These are not always available in the South African speech pathology experience, and consequently it is not yet clear how distance intervention might fit into service provision. It also appears that more time is needed for effective distance intervention with the Lidcombe Program. However, these issues need to be addressed, because many of the families needing help live in areas where there are no services, therapy resources are usually restricted to the main cities, and financial limitations make travel impossible for many.

Conclusion

At this stage, any conclusions about the use of the Lidcombe Program within the South African context can only be tentative, as there has not been sufficient time to assess its efficacy. There have, however, been gratifying preliminary results and much expressed interest by clinicians, both encouraging signs for the program's use in this country. Already the effect of this approach on treatment of the young child has become evident in the way that stuttering is viewed. More clinicians are prepared to treat young children who stutter and to learn about this method, and more parents are expressing satisfaction with the therapy process. Although this program has been introduced only recently to South Africa, it has already produced a definite shift in terms of both teaching and clinical work. Hopefully research will follow this positive trend.

Speech clinicians in South Africa are a small group. They qualify as speech–language clinicians and audiologists, and have to intervene with many kinds of communication problems in a country facing many social challenges. Demands exist for this limited number of clinicians to provide the best therapy to the most children with the minimum resources at their command. It is gratifying that the introduction of the Lidcombe Program has interested more clinicians in this field than before, and revitalized the concept of providing effective stuttering therapy with young children.

As noted previously, the minority of South Africans live in First World conditions, and can be thought of as having similar facilities and priorities as people in most other Western nations. However, most of the people, many rural but others living in urban areas, are economically and socially disadvantaged, and these function in Third World conditions. Our conclusions, therefore, will touch on each of these scenarios, beginning with the less privileged community.

As mentioned previously, there are many practical problems in implementing the Lidcombe Program with children and parents for whom even basic needs are not always met. A culture of poverty, joblessness, and poor living conditions makes for often insurmountable difficulties. Language and cultural differences further complicate the situation. Therefore, it does not seem tenable that therapy for many young stuttering children will be available or effective. For the more privileged group of South Africa, however, the situation appears similar to that of other Western countries. Clinicians have shown interest in the Lidcombe Program, and several have embraced it with enthusiasm. Parents, too, have found their involvement in the intervention program gratifying.

In South Africa the Lidcombe Program has been introduced into a speech pathology culture that has a much different background from that in which the treatment was developed. Traditionally, clinicians in South Africa have insisted that parents ignore the child's stuttering and that therapy concentrate on helping the parents to reduce stresses impinging on the child. The change from these methods to those of the Lidcombe Program is extreme. The introduction of this approach requires that clinicians make a radical shift in their thinking. South African clinicians have always embraced new ideas, however, and this holds positive promise for use of the program.

A matter of concern is selective usage of some aspects of the program. What seems to be occurring in South Africa is that elements of the Lidcombe Program are being used without regard for the entire program as it has been developed. There seems to be a potential danger that clinicians will use some features of the program, and try to fit it into their own eclectic approach. In this way, a watered-down version of the treatment might be used, and its efficacy diminished. Until research identifies which elements of the program are essential, it is important that it be used in its entirety, as it has been developed.

Despite the many challenges inherent in the South African context, clinicians strive to meet them and welcome innovative approaches such as that of the Lidcombe Program, whose practitioners stress the challenge that "therapy is problem solving." Professional workers in South Africa might have more problems to face than those in other countries but, together with support from colleagues all over the world, feel that their quests are rewarding and exciting. It is hoped that our experiences will be of value to workers in other countries with similar diversities of social structure, language, and culture.

Having been involved in the stuttering for many years, starting from 1954, and having been conversant with many of the new waves of treatment theory and practice over the last four decades, we welcome the empirically based Lidcombe Program. We are privileged to be involved in its implementation in South Africa, and hope that our work may add to the body of knowledge about this creative and exciting intervention with the young child who stutters.

References

Bloodstein, O. (1986). Semantics and beliefs. In G. H. Shames & H. Rubin (Eds.), *Stuttering then and now* (pp. 130– 139). Columbus, OH: Merrill.

Bluemel, C. S. (1935). *Stammering and allied disorders*. New York: Macmillan.

Costello, J. M. (1984). Treatment of the young chronic stutterer: Managing fluency. In R. F. Curlee & W. H. Perkins (Eds.), *Nature and treatment of stuttering: New directions* (pp. 375–395). San Diego: College-Hill Press.

Gregory, H. H., & Hill, D. (1980). Stuttering therapy for children. *Seminars in Speech, Language and Hearing, 1*, 351–363.

Harrison, E., Wilson, L., & Onslow, M. (1999). Distance intervention for early stuttering with the Lidcombe Programme. *Advances in Speech Language Pathology, 1*, 31–36.

Hayhow, R., Kingston, M., & Ledzion, R. (1998). The use of clinical measures in the Lidcombe Programme for children who stutter. *International Journal of Language & Communication Disorders, 33*, 364–369.

Ingham, R. J. (1984). *Stuttering and behavior therapy: Current status and experimental foundations*. San Diego: College-Hill Press.

Johnson, W. (1955). *Stuttering in children and adults*. Minneapolis: University of Minnesota Press.

Jones, M., Onslow, M., Harrison, E., & Packman, A. (2000). Treating stuttering in young children: Predicting treatment time in the Lidcombe Program. *Journal of Speech, Language, and Hearing Research, 43*, 1440–1450.

Levy, C., & Girson, J. (2001). The Lidcombe Program of early stuttering intervention: The South African perspective. In L. Wilson & S. Hewat (Eds.), *Proceedings of the 2001 Speech Pathology Australia National Conference* (pp. 65–71). Melbourne: Speech Pathology Australia.

Marks Wahlhaus, M. (1990). Stuttering: Can research unravel the riddle? *South African Journal of Communication Disorders, 37*, 35–38.

Ryan, B. P. (1979). Stuttering therapy in a framework of operant conditioning and programmed learning. In H. H. Gregory (Ed.), *Controversies about stuttering therapy* (pp. 129–173). Baltimore: University Park Press.

Shine, R. E. (1980). Direct management of the beginning stutterer. *Seminars in Speech and Language, 1*, 339–350.

Van Riper, C. (1973). *The treatment of stuttering*. Englewood Cliffs, NJ: Prentice Hall.

Wolpe, J. (1958). *Psychotherapy by reciprocal inhibition*. Stanford, CA: Stanford University Press.

Yairi, E., & Ambrose, N. (1992). A longitudinal study of stuttering in children: A preliminary report. *Journal of Speech and Hearing Research, 35*, 755–760.

Part V

Reflections

Chapter 16

Parents Talk About the Lidcombe Program

Mark Onslow, Joseph Attanasio, and Elisabeth Harrison

Much about the Lidcombe Program cannot be conveyed in the foregoing contents of this book. The focus of this chapter is what parents tell us about their experiences with the treatment.

The Lidcombe Program appears to be quite unique in speech pathology. That uniqueness relates to the fact that parents are empowered. They come to the clinician concerned that—as often happens—their children have a disorder with a rapid onset after a period of normal speech development. Then they conduct the treatment for their children themselves, and they ensure that treatment effects remain in place in the long term. We believe that this combination of factors, the bewildering and often distressing onset of the condition combined with its remediation by parents, gives rise to stories that are unique in clinical practice in this profession.

To convey some of the experiences of parents who helped treat their children using the Lidcombe Program, we randomly selected four mothers who had completed the Lidcombe Program or who were in the process of completing the program. The second author, who then interviewed them, was not expert in the treatment at the time and was a visitor to the Lidcombe clinics. What follows is a transcript of that interview. Minor editing was done to enhance readability, but this did not alter the content of the conversations.

JOSEPH: And she is happy?

ANN: Yeah, she loves going because she thinks that it is her special time and she is totally focused on it, and it is her special time with Margaret [her clinician], even though I am there and I have my little boy there with me. It's her special time and she gets rewards and she does what she wants to do. It's great, she loves it, she doesn't mind at all.

PAT: I have noticed how well and intelligently the therapist picks up on what the child likes and her interests and how they use that in therapy. And Sally loves it too.

MAY: Well, my son, we have actually finished the whole program. He is 5 and he started stuttering when he was 2½. Just quite suddenly out of the blue, really badly. And I started, um, we went to the baby health clinic first of all and they referred me to [a local hospital] speech therapy place there for a few months and he just sort of stagnated. It dropped, they improved it, but it just stabilized it and it wouldn't drop any further. She suggested that we come down here to Lidcombe, which we did. He loved coming down here too. He just gradually got down and down and then we got onto maintenance. We were on maintenance most of last year. And our last visit was just before Christmas. Very occasionally now I might hear a little hint of a stutter and pick him up on it. But now he has forgotten about bumpy words and he kind of looks at me as if to say, "What are you talking about?" So we have come a long way.

JOSEPH: Did you or the children experience any problems with the idea of the correction and the praise? How did they respond to that, having their stuttering corrected or their smooth speech praised?

SUE: I think with my daughter, it sort of depended on her moods. Sometimes I would correct her on it and she would say, and she would get really huffy with me and say "Oh I *am* talking properly." And then on other days it didn't affect her at all. Most of the time it didn't affect her, I must admit. But occasionally if I was correcting her a little bit too much one day, it was sort of like by the end of it she had had enough, and would tell me, "That's it, don't correct me any more, I have had it up to here." But most days I found the praise she loved, but most days correcting she handled it quite well actually. She knew that was part of the deal and she sort of accepted that was going to happen.

PAT: I found that Sally was such a talker anyway. I mean she wakes up in the morning talking and goes to bed at night talking. So getting her to talk wasn't a problem but sometimes, like your daughter, she would say "I *am* talking smoothly," depending on her mood. But there was no trouble getting her to talk; it was quite easy. And she was fine. We kept it to my husband and me correcting her and it wasn't a problem at all. We found there were differences between my husband and me. He couldn't be bothered sitting down for 15 minutes. He couldn't maintain that, so he would be more likely to just correct her at various times during the day and I would do sessions when we sat down for 15 or 20 minutes and that seemed to work quite well. And she accepted different methods from us. I don't know how it would have gone had we done the same thing.

JOSEPH: You had a similar experience?

MAY: Well, I think kids are like the rest of us, whatever you are praised for you do better at it as a result. And I think because the emphasis is on the praise but the correcting is in there so you sort of sneak the correcting in. But to me the praise is the main thing and they respond to that and therefore they take the correction when you point it out to them.

JOSEPH: So the correction became no problem?

MAY: They weren't for us, no. I can't really remember because it is a while now. I am sure we did have times when he did get a bit cranky too. But overall, because you are emphasizing the good aspects, you are saying "Good talking, good talking" a lot, then they keep trying. But at the same time they are being made aware of what they are saying, and how they are saying it. Which Matt was unaware of that until you point it out to them, I don't feel that they realize, some of them, that they are stuttering. And then at other times he knew that he was and he would be quite embarrassed, which is interesting.

PAT: Yes.

ANN: I tend to find that sometimes during the day, and if she has been at school during the day, she comes home and I haven't been saying—I have just been speaking—I haven't been saying, "That was great talking, that was smooth talking," she would come to me and say, "That was smooth talking, wasn't it Mummy?" And I will say, "Yes it was, it was great, that's really good." And I find that if I don't praise her enough, she tells me. She says to me, "That was good talking. That was smooth talking, wasn't it?"

SUE: I get exactly the same thing.

JOSEPH: So you are saying that the children are eagerly seeking out the praise?

ALL: Yeah, yeah.

ANN: They like the praise. And they remind you that "That was good talking, wasn't it?"

JOSEPH: And it allowed them to deal with the correction a bit more?

ALL: Yeah.

MAY: I think so.

ANN: And I also think it made them aware that they weren't stuttering. It made them aware that they were talking smoothly. And I think as the stutter becomes less, you don't praise them as much. You know like when it was high, you tend to forget a little bit. You don't forget—I don't know what the word is—you don't praise them as much as what it is when the severity is very high. I think they get used to the constant praise, praise, praise, and I think it makes them aware that they are not stuttering.

PAT: I never had the experience of a child who didn't know that she was stuttering. Mine knew so desperately that she was stuttering that she stopped talking. She was always very aware and it really inhibited her and she searched around for different—she always had a very well-developed vocabulary. So she would search around for different words because that was at her disposal. She was always very good with words, unlike her mother who is making a meal of this sentence! But she found it extraordinarily frustrating and she knew what was going on and it was very difficult and it was really awful.

SUE: My daughter was picked out actually by a little girl in the street, who asked, "Why does she talk so funny and why doesn't she talk properly?" And she said to me, "How come I don't speak properly?" and I said, "You do, you tell her that we are getting it fixed and that you speak very well for your age." And she was a little bit upset by that, that someone noticed that she didn't talk properly.

PAT: A next door neighbor said that she was a bad girl because she wasn't talking, that she was too lazy.

SUE: Yes, sort of like that, and that was a bit upsetting at the time and that was when we were waiting to get into the Lidcombe Program, and I kept thinking I hope this hurries soon, I hope it comes along soon, I can't stand this any longer for her because I really felt for her that day.

JOSEPH: Have things like that changed as a result of the program? You have talked about changes in the speech. Have there been changes in other aspects of the children's lives? Have they become more talkative again, teasing stopped, have there been other kinds of influences?

SUE: More confident. They become more confident just with themselves and speaking with other people. And just their sports, their activities. I found with my—my little girl is in year one this year, and last year the teacher said, "She is very quiet, I don't even know that I have her." I said, "Yeah, I know, that is what she is like. She is a very placid little thing." If you put her anywhere in the classroom, she will sit and you won't even know that she is there. But this year she is participating more. She is reading better, she is doing everything better, she is doing better at school.

JOSEPH: That's wonderful.

ALL: Mmm.

SUE: Yeah, I think it has improved her lifestyle. As you say, with everything. She will play with all the kids out on the street now and she has got no fear. For a while she was a bit frightened that someone would pick on her again. And now she just sort of is, like, with them all the time. Yeah. And is not bothered by it at all. And now sometimes I forget that she had a problem. When you are not hearing it all the time, you forget to praise. And she will come to me and say, "Did you hear what I just said? Wasn't that good?" And I will say, "That was excellent." And I thought, I must remember.

JOSEPH: So she is very proud of her accomplishments?

SUE: Oh very proud. Very proud, very proud. She thinks she is really good.

JOSEPH: As she is.

SUE: She is, she is really good.

JOSEPH: Have your children experienced some changes like that in other aspects in their lives?

PAT: Do you feel that way May?

MAY: Not so dramatically, probably because he was so young and it was corrected fairly quickly, we didn't have those kinds of problems.

JOSEPH: Okay. They were prevented from occurring.

MAY: Well, yeah, probably. Yes. Adults certainly noticed. Adults commented to me, "Oh isn't his speech improving" after we got into the program, "He is not stuttering near as much." But other children tended not to notice because we were mixing with young children at that stage as well.

SUE: I found that children from, like, playgroup, that were the same age as herself, didn't notice. They are so involved with themselves, they tend not to notice what other children are doing. But the children in our street are quite a few years older than her. She was 9, this little girl who tended to pick on my daughter's speech. Well, my daughter was 2 at the time, and I noticed that she wasn't speaking properly.

PAT: I had such a verbally precocious child that she would talk anywhere all the time. It didn't matter, when she was talking again, after she went through that stage of not saying very much at all and stopped reciting her books and poems. Then once she got over that and we started the program, she then would talk, whether she stuttered or not, she just talked. And that made it harder in some ways because she wasn't thinking about what she was saying. She was so busy trying to tell you something, it didn't matter whether she stuttered or not. I think it made the problem worse.

ANN: I just had one experience. This was in the playground a little while ago. I had one of her little friends come up to me, and this was a day when I picked her up from school and she was stuttering quite noticeably. And the little girl actually came up to me and said, "Why does she talk like that? Why does she talk so funny for?" And, you know, it sort of puts you on the spot. And you think, "She doesn't mean to, she can't help it." You know, some days are better than others. She didn't approach my child, she approached me.

SUE: I wish this little girl had approached me and not said it to her.

JOSEPH: Well, is it obvious that a lot of the responsibility is on you, with the clinician, with the staff people instructing you?

ALL: Yeah.

JOSEPH: What does that do for you, or what kind of difficulty does that give you, knowing that you have the responsibility of carrying out the program?

SUE: Well, it was not really a burden or a responsibility. Well, it was a responsibility but it was my decision to do it because I wanted her speech improved. So I didn't really look at it as if it was something really difficult to do. I just looked at it as this is what we have to do if we want you to speak smoothly.

MAY: We were told that they have had good success with it. And you think that it is worth trying.

ALL: Yeah.

MAY: It is worth trying. There was a fair chance that it would succeed. It is like anything you do if you can do it for your child.

SUE: You will do it.

MAY: This thing which is like a sickness with them, then you will do it.

PAT: I had some hesitancy over whether I was in fact doing it correctly.

ALL: Oh yeah.

PAT: That was something that I thought quite a lot about, particularly in the early stages. And, too, my husband and I virtually took it in turns, because of work commitments, in taking my daughter to therapy so there wasn't always that backup, or the luxury of going all the time for some consistency. Mind you, I think it helped her in the end because we both became proficient at the treatment. But I did find I was quite concerned whether I was doing it correctly and the impact I would be having if I was doing it wrong. You know, what were the implications.

SUE: I had the same thing, feeling, at first: "Oh, gee, did I say the right thing, was I supposed to correct her then? Oh well, I'll praise her a couple of times now to make up for that correction."

MAY: But after a while it sort of becomes second nature, doesn't it?

SUE: Yeah.

ALL: Yeah.

JOSEPH: And you could bring these problems along to the next visit?

ALL: Yes.

MAY: And they were always encouraging, too.

ALL: Oh very.

ANN: You thought you were doing a good job. That is the first thing that they do. They talk to the child. And ask you how you are going. But then they sit down, well this is what Margaret does with me. She lets my kids sit down and my little boy sits down and says, "Have you got this, have you got this, have you got this?" It is my daughter who is having the therapy, and he has a list of all the things that she has to bring for it. And Margaret says, "I am just going to have a chat with mum now," which I find very good too, because then I can say if things are going well or if it's not going well or what's happening. And they always allow that time for you too, which is good.

MAY: In a sense the visit is as much, well, as much for me as it was for them.

SUE: Oh, Liz is the same. You have half and half with her. There is a percentage of the time that you are in there that she actually speaks to you and asks how you are going. And that's when you can say to her, "I have said this and I have done that. Should I have said something a little differently?" or "What would I do in this situation?" And then she would tell you, you know. So it is very good, they are very good.

PAT: And I found in-between times, I felt free to ring up and say, "My daughter all of a sudden has got worse."

JOSEPH: So you can call.

ALL: Oh yes.

MAY: They always encourage you to ring if you have any queries or problems, which is very reassuring. Which is good, especially in the early stages.

ALL: Oh yes.

JOSEPH: That's great! Is there anything else?

SUE: I am just so glad I did it. You know, had I have listened to so many people that used to tell me, "All children stutter, oh I remember mine stuttered, oh they will grow out of it."

ANN: It's just a phase . . .

SUE: . . . it is just a phase. I am glad that I did it when I did it.

PAT: I tell people that the only thing children grow out of is their clothes. You have to do something about it. I am really pleased.

JOSEPH: Well thank you.

Chapter 17

Issues

Ann Packman

More then 10 years have passed since the first published report (Onslow, Costa, & Rue, 1990) of the behavioral treatment for stuttering that was later to be known as the Lidcombe Program. As is clear from this text, much has happened since then. The program is now widely accepted in Australia (see Chapter 11) and is also used in a number of other countries around the world, such as the United Kingdom, Canada, New Zealand, South Africa, Holland, and most recently the United States. The development over the last 10 years of this direct, parent-delivered program has raised a number of interesting issues. The program has not been accepted in all countries, for example, without question or controversy. This chapter explores some of these issues, and some others as well. Most have already been addressed to some extent in Chapter 3. The issues can be seen as falling into four groups: cultural, procedural, theoretical, and empirical.

Cultural Issues

Over the last 10 years, those of us who have presented Lidcombe Program workshops and conference papers internationally have occasionally encountered negative reactions to the program (e.g., Cook & Rustin, 1997; Hayhow, 1997; Onslow, O'Brian, & Harrison, 1997). At first we thought this was a cultural issue and we considered the possibility that the Lidcombe Program simply did not translate to countries other than Australia. Perhaps, we thought, the program was somehow a product of the well-known trait of Australians to "call a spade a spade," and that the directness of the program is uniquely compatible with the apparently pragmatic Australian character. Perhaps other cultures might simply find such a direct approach to stuttering, and indeed to children, unpalatable (for a discussion of cultural issues in stuttering, see Attanasio, Onslow, & Menzies, 1996).

In retrospect, this is probably only partly true. As is clear from Chapter 2, the professional and scientific environment in Australia in the 1980s was indeed quite unique, steeped as it was in the influence of behavior therapy. That environment provided the conditions necessary for the Lidcombe Program to develop—and flourish. But, as is clear from this text, in time clinicians from other countries around the world have become interested in the program, some even enthusiastically, and many now report that they are quite comfortable using it.

It took a while for us to realize that we had contributed at least in part to early scepticism about the program. Looking back, it seems that our early writings about the program conveyed the impression, quite unwittingly, that the treatment is programmed and inflexible and that children who participate are submitted to unremitting parental negativity and attention to speech. We were amazed when clinicians who attended workshops and presentations told us that, when they saw our video footage of the program, they realized quite the opposite is true. We came to understand that our professional writings had failed to convey the essence of the program, namely that it is a positive experience for the child and the family. Children love the program, and so do parents (see Chapter 16). Children participate in enjoyable activities, and their comments frequently convey that they are pleased with themselves when they find they can talk without stuttering. In turn, parents report that they feel empowered to help their children because, as therapists, they play an active role in treatment and participate with the clinician in decisions about how the program is implemented. We had assumed that readers around the world would understand all that, just as we understood it. How wrong we were.

Nonetheless, interesting issues are arising in relation to the Lidcombe Program as it is used in other cultures. The chapters in this text dealing with the use of the program in other countries highlight a number of these issues. Using the program in a language other than English, for example, raises interesting issues. As reported by the Canadians who are now using the program extensively in French, finding French equivalents for much of the terminology has apparently not been easy (see Chapter 13). Only recently, a clinician from another culture distant both geographically and culturally from Australia remarked that praising children is not commonplace in that culture. The clinician said that when children participate in the program, they are puzzled as to why their parents comment on how well they are speaking. And the challenges of delivering the Lidcombe Program in a country such as South Africa, as described in Chapter 15, are enormous.

We look forward to more exchanges about cultural differences as more clinicians from other cultures use the program, particularly in languages other than English. Perhaps the program may in time act as a cultural bridge, leading to the sharing of stories of how the program works—or not, as the case may be—in different cultures.

Procedural Issues

The Use of Operant Methods (Verbal Contingencies)

One objection we sometimes encounter is that the Lidcombe Program involves operant methods. The very term conjures up visions of laboratories and experimenters in white coats using electric shocks. Of course, those visions have no place in the Lidcombe Program. The operant procedures in the Lidcombe Program are verbal in nature, they are not programmed, and the ratio of reinforcement to punishment is always *at least* 5:1 (see Chapter 6). The terminology of operant methodology, such as *reinforcement* and *punishment*, also conjures up visions of perfunctory and unfeeling manipulation of behavior. Of course, once converted to user-friendly terms, such as praise and requests for self-correction, or even just contingencies, the terminology loses its negative valence and becomes much more acceptable.

Yet, the procedures in the Lidcombe Program are indeed operant, and in operant parlance the contingencies in the program are indeed reinforcers and punishers. When given in a treatment program, contingencies (events that follow a designated behavior or, more accurately, class of behaviors) are regarded as reinforcing if they are thought likely to increase the frequency or duration of the behavior. Thus, when a parent comments on or praises the child for stutter-free speech, it is done with the expectancy that the child will produce more of it. Similarly, contingencies are regarded as punishing when they are thought likely to decrease the frequency or duration of a behavior. Thus, when a parent comments on or otherwise draws the child's attention to stuttering, it is done with the expectancy that the child will stutter less. There is plenty of clinical and laboratory research to indicate that stuttering can be controlled in this way (see Chapter 3; Ingham, 1984; Prins & Hubbard, 1988). However, these contingencies can only be regarded as truly reinforcing and punishing if stuttering in fact reduces. That is why measurement of stuttering is critical to the conduct of the Lidcombe Program. If stuttering is not reducing, then the contingencies are not having the desired effect. This may be due to one or a number of factors, including that the contingencies thought to be reinforcing are not reinforcing at all. For example, occasional parental praise such as "Good talking" will be reinforcing for most children, but not for all. The clinician needs to find out if this is the case, and modify the contingencies accordingly.

There are other implications, too, of using operant methods with young children who stutter. The first is that the operant procedures in the Lidcombe Program involve systematically drawing attention to stuttering, albeit in a palatable way. In our experience, parents and clinicians in Australia occasionally say that they feel uncomfortable doing this. However, as is apparent from reports in other chapters, this is more the case in other countries, and there is no doubt that there is still a pervasive feeling, presumably a legacy of an earlier theoretical view, that parents must not talk about stuttering in front of the child and that drawing attention to stuttering will make the disorder worse. Of course, drawing attention to stuttering *in the context of the Lidcombe Program* does not distress children and does not make stuttering worse. Indeed, the program would not have survived for at least 10 years if that were the case. The codicil here is that the implementation of these operant procedures must always be supervised by an experienced clinician who checks each week that the program remains a positive experience for the child and family.

Another problem some people have with operant procedures, at least as they are incorporated into the Lidcombe Program, is that the parent applies verbal contingencies to the *way* the child talks; that is, the parent provides contingencies for speech that is stutter-free and speech that is stuttered. This is not, of course, the advice typically given to parents of a child of this age to stimulate language development. Clinicians, and more often university academicians, have suggested that attending to *how* a child speaks is somehow incompatible with the sorts of strategies that clinicians and parents use to extend children's language. It is felt that giving praise for talking is somehow aberrant, as children should be reinforced for linguistic content rather than speech production. Our response to this is that the two are entirely compatible. The verbal contingencies of the Lidcombe Program are delivered during conversational exchanges, and parents learn very quickly how to deliver contingencies while at the same time engaging the child appropriately in conversation.

In the past, clinicians sometimes said to us that they were uncomfortable with the very idea of praising stutter-free speech and correcting stuttering. They reported that they felt that this procedure passed judgment on the child's speech performance. However, they were usually reassured when they found that the clinician ensures that parental verbal contingencies convey knowledge of results rather than approval or disapproval (see Chapter 6). For example, nonjudgmental comments such as "That was smooth talking," "No bumpy words there," and "I didn't hear any stutters that time" convey facts. Those comments should predominate in the reinforcement of stutter-free speech, with judgmental comments such as "Good boy!" and "Good talking!" used sparingly. The same applies to verbal contingencies for stuttering, which should consist *only* of knowledge of results, such as "That was a bit bumpy," or requests for repair, such as "Can you say that word smoothly?" Contingencies for stuttering should never be aversive or punitive, or convey to the child in any way that the parent is displeased (see Chapter 6).

It is worth noting that treatments for other communication disorders in children, such as phonological disorders, also involve providing knowledge of results and even praise for correct productions. However, these treatments do not seem to prompt the same disquiet as is sometimes the case with stuttering treatment. Again, this disquiet in regard to stuttering can be traced back to the view that drawing attention to stuttering will make the condition worse—a legacy of the diagnosogenic theory that held such sway in previous decades (see Chapter 3).

Finally, training parents to do the treatment also involves the application of behavioral principles, including contingencies. The clinician models the delivery of treatment in the clinic and then requests the parent to do it. The clinician reinforces the parent's behavior when it conforms sufficiently to the model and draws attention to, or corrects, the parent's delivery of the treatment when it does not.

The Treatment Appears To Be Simple

Another objection to the program encountered occasionally is that it appears to be simple, and is therefore inappropriate for a disorder that is currently viewed by many as multifactorial and therefore complex (e.g., see Cook & Rustin, 1997). However, stuttering can be viewed as both complex and simple according to one's perspective. It is true that many factors influence stuttering and that it is therefore multidimensional in nature. And there is no doubt that the behaviors of stuttering may become complex, as the topography of stuttering changes and becomes idiosyncratic over time. However, the first signs of stuttering are almost always syllable repetitions, suggesting that the factor or factors underlying stuttering, may in fact be quite simple (Attanasio, Onslow, & Packman, 1998) although not necessarily simple to identify. Outcome studies of the Lidcombe Program suggest that the apparent complexity of the behaviors of stuttering and the fact that no two people who stutter do so in exactly the same way are immaterial. The parent is not required to identify different types of stuttering, nor is the program implemented differently for different stuttering behaviors. Stuttering is the response class, regardless of topography. This is not to say that *severity* of stuttering is immaterial. Indeed, as has been made clear in this text, stuttering rate is critical in individualizing the way the program is implemented, not only across children but also during the course of treatment for each child.

It will also be obvious from reading this text that the program is not a one-size-fits-all treatment. Although the essential features of the program are stipulated in this guide, the text also indicates that the implemetation of those essential features must be tailored for individual children. It is hoped that, after finishing this text, the reader will be in no doubt that there are as many ways to implement the Lidcombe Program as there are families who participate in it.

Parents Implement the Treatment

The Lidcombe Program is delivered by parents in the child's everyday environment. This involves what is seen by some clinicians as a role reversal (Packman & Onslow, 2000). Clinicians may not be accustomed, in stuttering treatments at least, to handing over responsibility for delivering treatment to a parent. Of course, it is important to stipulate here that we are referring to direct treatment; parents have for decades been instructed to alter various aspects of the child's environment in indirect treatments for stuttering.

However, expecting parents to implement direct treatment, as occurs in the Lidcombe Program, is quite another matter. Clinicians are sometimes apprehensive about doing this, fearing, among other things, that the parent will not do the treatment correctly. This fear is usually countered when the clinician understands how to monitor the treatment carefully, by observing the parent conducting the treatment in the clinic and, if necessary, by having the parent bring from home tape recordings of the treatment sessions.

Another unique feature of the program is that the clinician and parent work as a team, making joint decisions about how the program proceeds. The parent is the expert on the child, and the clinician is the expert on stuttering. Mutual respect and cooperation are required for this collaboration to work. Some clinicians find this sharing of the role of expert unsettling at first. Parents may feel this way also. In most Western societies health consumers are conditioned to expect professionals to provide a diagnosis, prescribe the treatment, and carry out any required procedures. Some parents are more comfortable in the role of patient, or health service consumer, than that of therapist.

Theoretical Issues

The Lidcombe Program is a behavioral treatment and was developed empirically rather than from a particular theoretical view of the nature or cause of stuttering (see Chapter 2). It evolved from laboratory and other findings about the variables that control stuttering. The influence of behavior therapy on the program is apparent in the reliance on the scientific method and exemplified in the use of measurement throughout the program.

This atheoretical approach means, however, that the program can be seen to be at odds with a popular current view on early stuttering. This view is that stuttering is a multifactorial disorder, and that treatment should be driven by this. For example, the Demands and Capacities model (DCM; Adams, 1990; Gottwald & Starkweather, 1995; Starkweather, 1987, 1997; Starkweather & Givens-Ackerman, 1997; Starkweather & Gottwald, 1990; Starkweather, Gottwald, & Halfond, 1990), which is the predominant multifactorial view of early stuttering, has influenced much current thinking about the nature of stuttering and early intervention.

The DCM states that children start to stutter when their capacity for fluent speech is insufficient to meet the demands to produce it. According to the DCM, a child's capacity for fluency depends on speech motor development, language development, social and emotional functioning, and cognitive development. The demands on those capacities include time pressure, innate and environmental pressure to use increasingly more complex language, high levels of excitement and anxiety, and parental demands for increased cognitive functioning. For stuttering to occur, it is not necessary for there to be excessive demands or a deficit in capacities. According to the DCM, the etiology of stuttering is different for each child depending on the unique configuration of these demands and capacities (Starkweather & Givens-Ackerman, 1997). The approach to therapy generated by the DCM is to redress, for each child, what is judged to be the discrepancy between the child's capacity for fluency and the demands placed on that capacity. Consequently, therapy involves, among other things, reducing any communicative demands in the child's everyday environment that the clinician hypothesizes have some functional or causal association with the child's stuttering.

A logical prediction of the DCM is that stuttering will get worse if demands for fluency increase. Yet stuttering improves with the Lidcombe Program, a treatment that clearly imposes demands on the child to speak without stuttering. This should not be taken to mean that the demands for fluency made by parents in the Lidcombe Program are delivered in an imperious manner or that children perceive parental verbal contingencies as "demanding," in the way this term is typically used. But the fact remains that in the Lidcombe Program the parent draws the child's attention to stuttering in everyday speaking situations, conveys to the child that he or she should try to speak without stuttering, and reinforces stutter-free speech when the child produces it. In addition, altering the communicative styles of other people in the child's environment and reducing possible stressors in the child's life are not part of the Lidcombe Program. Indeed, the goal of the Lidcombe Program is for children to speak without stuttering in their natural environment, *despite* the rough-and-tumble and communicative demands of everyday life. The approach of the Lidcombe Program, then, is diametrically opposed to that of DCM-based treatment, which advocates reducing demands for fluency rather than increasing them.

In a recent forum about the DCM (Bernstein Ratner, 2000; Curlee, 2000; Kelly, 2000; Manning, 2000a, 2000b; Siegel, 2000; Starkweather & Gottwald, 2000; Yaruss, 2000), Siegel raised a number of concerns about the validity of the DCM and its implications for the treatment of children who stutter. As noted by Siegel, there has been little critical assessment of the model, despite the fact that it has been referred to in the stuttering literature for decades. With the exception of Starkweather and Gottwald, the respondents agreed—to varying extents—with the concerns raised by Siegel, and some raised further concerns of their own; however, not one thought the model should be discarded. Yet evidence from outcome studies of the Lidcombe Program cannot, it seems, be reconciled with the DCM. In fact, this evidence is a direct challenge to the DCM. The Lidcombe Program would not have survived so long if it made stuttering worse, as the DCM predicts.

Empirical Issues

The Lidcombe Program is influenced by the principles of behavior therapy, and consequently incorporates aspects of the scientific method. There is, therefore, a reliance on empiricism; for example, the collection of stuttering measures is an integral part of the program and clinical decisions are guided by them (see Chapter 5). Furthermore, one of the notable features of the development of the Lidcombe Program is that there is considerable empirical evidence with which to assess its worth as a treatment. This evidence relates both to outcomes of the program and to the therapy process itself. At the time of writing, a controlled clinicial trial is under way (see Chapter 14) that will provide evidence for a third area of interest, namely the effectiveness of the program.

While research into these three areas continues, there are at least two other questions that interest us and that invite empirical answers: (1) Why does the Lidcombe Program work? and (2) Are all components of the program necessary to its effectiveness?

Why Does the Lidcombe Program Work?

People often ask why the Lidcombe Program works (see Onslow et al., 1997). This question is usually prompted by the fact that, as discussed previously, the treatment is not theory driven. Those who think that treatment should accord with a theoretical position on the cause of stuttering may feel that they cannot make sense of a treatment that is without theoretical underpinnings.

Our usual response to that question is that, at the present time, it is sufficient to have empirical evidence that the treatment works. Of course, that is not the only criterion for selecting a treatment. A treatment must also be safe and without unwanted side effects, it must be a positive experience for the child and family, it must have social validity, and its effects must be apparent across speaking contexts and over time.

All that we know is that children speak without stuttering when environmental consequences are applied in a systematic fashion to both stutter-free speech and stuttering. We cannot explain why this happens. Nor is it necessary to explain why this happens. If the treatment works and is otherwise acceptable, then an explanation is not required. Nonetheless, the question of why the Lidcombe Program works is not without theoretical interest.

For us, however, speculation about why the program works will be fueled by empiricism. In other words, if we want to explain why it works, we would look to evidence generated by research into the program.

Some recent research is interesting in this regard. In attempts to show that the program is safe, a number of preliminary studies have investigated whether the program results in unusual or unwanted effects. No such effects were found in language usage, speech acoustics, or psychological adjustment (see Chapter 4). The first two findings are of interest because they suggest that children do not achieve stutter-free speech by altering either the way they use language or the way they produce speech. In other words, the findings suggest that these factors probably do *not* contribute to the reductions of stuttering that occur with the program, although, of course, generalizing from these very preliminary negative findings is unwise. At the present time, then, the question of why the Lidcombe Program works remains unanswered. We will continue to look for clues in research findings as they emerge, although it must be said that an empirical explanation may elude us. The program may work because it simply teaches children another way of talking—a way that does not include stuttering. It is possible that such learning may occur in young children without any detectable changes to linguistic factors such as grammatical complexity, or to motor factors such as speech rate, articulation, and other aspects of speech production.

Are All Components of the Program Necessary to Its Effectiveness?

The Lidcombe Program was developed as a package, and it is by no means clear that all the components of the package are essential to the program's effectiveness. This is an important issue, because nonessential components could be dispensed with, thus simplifying the program and increasing its efficiency.

The treatment agents incorporated into the program are verbal contingencies for stuttering and stutter-free speech. As discussed, considerable evidence from laboratory and treatment studies indicates that these contingencies control stuttering. Indeed, that is why they are included in the program. However, it is not known that both are critical to the control of stuttering, at least in the context of the Lidcombe Program. It is possible, for example, that contingencies for stuttering add no more to treatment effects than contingencies for stutter-free speech. If that were known to be the case, then the contingencies for stuttering could be dispensed with. That would be positive development.

Other components of the program also may be dispensable. Parental severity ratings were incorporated into the program primarily because of the known variability of stuttering across situations. It is common sense to measure stuttering in the real world, where the problem occurs, as well as in the clinic. Although clinicians report that they think parental measures of stuttering are critical to the program, that has never been shown to be the case. In short, this study will determine whether contingencies for stuttering and parental measures of stuttering contribute to treatment effectiveness. Of course, a measurable contribution to effectiveness is not the only criterion for including various features of treatment.

Conclusion

The Lidcombe Program can be seen as an entity in itself, or it can be seen as a model for delivering a treatment agent. That treatment agent is parental verbal contingencies for stuttering and stutter-free speech. Our program of research is trying to establish whether other models of service delivery might also be effective. One alternative model is telehealth (see Chapter 11). Replacing weekly clinic visits with communication using information technology would make a significant contribution to making the program more accessible to rural and remotely located families. Research into developing other models of service delivery is also under way.

References

Adams, M. R. (1990). The demands and capacity model: 1. Theoretical elaborations. *Journal of Fluency Disorders, 15*, 135–141.

Attanasio, J., Onslow, M., & Menzies, R. (1996). Australian and American perspectives on early stuttering. *Australian Journal of Human Communication Disorders, 24*, 55–61.

Attanasio, J., Onslow, M., & Packman, A. (1998). Representativeness reasoning and the search for the origins of stuttering: A return to basic observations. *Journal of Fluency Disorders, 23*, 265–277.

Bernstein Ratner, N. (2000). Performance or capacity, the model still requires definitions and boundaries it doesn't have. *Journal of Fluency Disorders, 25*, 337–348.

Cook, F., & Rustin, L. (1997). Commentary on the Lidcombe Programme of early stuttering intervention. *European Journal of Disorders of Communication, 32*, 250–258.

Curlee, R. F. (2000). Demands and capacities versus demands and performance. *Journal of Fluency Disorders, 25*, 329–336.

Gottwald, S. R., & Starkweather, C. W. (1995). Fluency intervention for preschoolers and their families in the public schools. *Language, Speech, and Hearing Services in Schools, 26*, 117–126.

Hayhow, R. (1997). Commentary on Onslow, O'Brian, and Harrison. *European Journal of Disorders of Communication, 32*, 258–266.

Ingham, R. J. (1984). *Stuttering and behavior therapy: Current status and experimental foundations*. San Diego: College-Hill Press.

Kelly, E. (2000). Modeling stuttering etiology: Clarifying levels of description and measurement. *Journal of Fluency Disorders, 25*, 359–368.

Manning, W. H. (2000a). Appeal of the demands and capacities model: Conclusions. *Journal of Fluency Disorders, 25*, 377–383.

Manning, W. H. (2000b). The demands and capacities model. *Journal of Fluency Disorders, 25*, 317–319.

Onslow, M., Costa, L., & Rue, S. (1990). Direct early intervention with stuttering: Some preliminary data. *Journal of Speech and Hearing Disorders, 55*, 405–416.

Onslow, M., O'Brian, S., & Harrison, E. (1997). The Lidcombe Programme of early stuttering intervention: Methods and issues. *European Journal of Disorders of Communication, 32*, 231–250.

Packman, A., & Onslow, M. (2000). The Lidcombe Program for early stuttering: The old and the new. In H.-G. Bosshardt, J. S. Yaruss, & H. F. M. Peters (Eds.), *Fluency disorders: Theory, research, treatment and self-help* (pp. 266–270). Nijmegen, The Netherlands: Nijmegen University Press.

Prins, D., & Hubbard, C. P. (1988). Response contingent stimuli and stuttering: Issues and implications. *Journal of Speech and Hearing Research, 31*, 696–709.

Siegel, G. M. (2000). Demands and capacities or demands and performance? *Journal of Fluency Disorders, 25*, 321–327.

Starkweather, C. W. (1987). *Fluency and stuttering*. Englewood Cliffs, NJ: Prentice Hall.

Starkweather, C. W. (1997). Therapy for younger children. In R. F. Curlee & G. M. Siegel (Eds.), *Nature and treatment of stuttering: New directions* (2nd ed., pp. 257–279). Boston: Allyn & Bacon.

Starkweather, C. W., & Givens-Ackerman, J. (1997). *Stuttering*. Austin, TX: PRO-ED.

Starkweather, C. W., & Gottwald, S. R. (1990). The demands and capacities model: II. Clinical applications. *Journal of Fluency Disorders, 15*, 143–157.

Starkweather, C. W., & Gottwald, S. R. (2000). The demands and capacities model: Response to Siegel. *Journal of Fluency Disorders, 25*, 369–375.

Starkweather, C. W., Gottwald, S. R., & Halfond, M. M. (1990). *Stuttering prevention: A clinical method*. Englewood Cliffs, NJ: Prentice Hall.

Yaruss, J. S. (2000). The role of performance in the demands and capacities model. *Journal of Fluency Disorders, 25*, 347–358.

Chapter 18

Some Observations and Reflections

Joseph Attanasio

My task in this chapter is to offer a closing summation of the text. Rather than merely summarizing what has been stated quite clearly in each of the chapters, however, I have chosen to reflect broadly on what is contained in the text and on the Lidcombe Program itself. The reflections are at times personal and at times professional.

A New Jersey Yank in Lidcombe, Australia's Court

The origins of the Lidcombe Program may be found in the Midwest of the United States in the early 1970s, as Mark Onslow reports in Chapter 2 of this text, but it took a fresh breeze from Australia to clean out the cobwebs that coated the then contemporary thinking on the treatment of early stuttering. My first encounter with Onslow, his colleagues, and the Lidcombe Program, was when I read an article published in one of the American research journals (Onslow, Costa, & Rue, 1990). Although I was a mature professional clinician and academician at the time (I believe that is a fair self-description) and well read in the field of stuttering, I sat reading that article with eyes wide open and jaw dropped. Here in print was the bold implication that young children, indeed very young children, who stutter (it was equally bold at the time to use "stutter" rather than "disfluent" when referring to young children) could be treated directly, openly, and freely. Finally, I thought, someone is putting into print a point of view about stuttering that I long held but could not support by recourse to the published literature. Well, there was some published literature to point to (e.g., Culatta, 1976; Martin, Kuhl, & Haroldson, 1972; Prins & Ingham, 1983), but for some reason it was the article that I was reading at that moment that caused me to celebrate. Today's speech–language pathologists may not be able to understand my excitement or why what I was reading was somewhat revolutionary because many speech–language pathologists currently in practice have not grown up, as I did, in the diagnosogenic era. Anyone unfamiliar with Wendell Johnson's work ought to read up a bit so that the full implications of the Australian breeze that blew out of the Lidcombe suburb of Sydney can be appreciated. In Chapter 3 of this text, Barry Guitar provides excellent overviews of the history of early stuttering treatment, Johnson's diagnosogenic theory, and the currently fashionable but problematic Demands and Capacities treatment model. Several other chapters also provide historical background.

I decided that I had to contact Professor Onslow. I wrote to congratulate him on the article—I did suggest one weakness in the methodology—and he wrote a cordial letter back. Our correspondence and collaboration continues to this day, including my visit to the Australian Stuttering Research Centre in 1996 and Mark Onslow and Ann Packman's subsequent visit to my university in New Jersey.

My visit to Australia led me to believe that the approach to early stuttering intervention reflected in the Lidcombe Program is an offspring of what might be called an Australian professional culturalism—that is, a professional and cultural outlook different than what was the case in the United States and little influenced by the diagnosogenic theory and its effect on American speech–language pathology. This outlook provided the spark for a long-needed change in the ways we viewed and treated early stuttering (see Attanasio, Onslow, & Menzies, 1996, for a full explication of these points). I had become a New Jersey Yank in Lidcombe, Australia.

It is my sense that American speech–language pathologists, those who treat stuttering and those who remain timid about its treatment, are not yet fully aware of the Lidcombe Program. The outlook, however, is quite promising. This Clinician's Guide, which contains contributions from Americans, and the collaborations that Mark Onslow, Ann Packman, and their colleagues have with American academicians and clinicians, will have a positive impact on the treatment of early stuttering in the United States. That impact has already been felt and changes in thinking have already occurred. The same may be said for the worldwide context.

On the Issue of Models

If the reader steps back a moment from the details of the Lidcombe Program described in this guide and considers the treatment on a conceptual level, it will become clear that it is a true interactionist, or better yet, transactional, model of intervention in which treatment factors have a dynamic and reciprocal relationship and interact with one another to reduce or eliminate stuttering. Changes in one factor produce changes in the other factors. Hubbell's (1981) description of a transactional model in his discussion of causation in children's language disorders may be applied to the dynamics of the treatment concepts within the Lidcombe Program. Hubbell (1981) wrote,

> At any point in time the child's constitution is in a certain state, indicated by C1. In a parallel fashion, the environment is also in a certain state at the same time, indicated by E1. Both child and environment respond to each other, and thus change each other and are themselves changed. Consequently, at a later time (indicated by C2 and E2), each is now different. They are still influencing each other, so that at a still later time, both are different again. The process continues throughout life. Thus, environments influence children, but at the same time children influence environments. The net result is that children alter the environments that affect them and vice versa, in continuing reciprocal fashion. (p. 112)

Hubbell (1981) incorporated environmental and constitutional factors in his explanation of a transactional model. The primary factors in the Lidcombe Program are (1) the instances of the appropriate response-contingent stimulation (RCS) provided by the parent in response to (2) the stuttered or stutter-free speech of the child. The context, timing, and nature of RCS are dependent on the child's stuttered or stutter-free speech and they change according to the kind of speech the child produces. In turn, the child's speech is changed as a result of the RCS. This interaction between the factors continues in a dynamically reciprocal fashion throughout the program. True interactionist or transactional treatment models must delineate those factors that are the targets of intervention, specify how those factors interact, and utilize data-based clinical measures to assess outcomes (Attanasio, 2000). All of those elements are incorporated within the Lidcombe Program and are outlined in the text. To my knowledge, this characterization of the program as transactional has not been made explicit in previous descriptions.

It might be instructive here to revisit the Demands and Capacities model (DCM), and comment briefly on its claim to being an interactionist model, so that the truly interactional or transactional nature of the Lidcombe Program described previously can be better appreciated. Although the DCM is more comprehensive and complex than a linear model and although it rejects single-variable or single-factor explanations of stuttering, it becomes apparent when it is examined more closely that, despite the fact that it combines the two factors of nature and nurture, those factors are in a linear and unidirectional relationship to one another. In a real sense, such models as the DCM are misnamed as interactionist. They are best viewed, I suggest, as complex versions of a simple linear unidirectional model; the DCM is such a model. In actuality, the DCM is only saying that the environment has an influence on fluency and that the child's constitution has an influence on fluency. On the other hand, models that are truly interactionist illustrate the ways in which factors (e.g., constitution and environment) affect one another or are changed by one another.

The DCM fails as an interactionist model because it does nothing more than catalog those constitutional factors on one hand and those environmental factors on the other that have been implicated in stuttering. It suggests that a child stutters as a result of a capacity for fluency that is not up to the demands of the child's environment or, conversely, a child stutters because the demands of the environment overtax the child's capacity for fluency. The absolute levels of that capacity or of the demands of that environment are not at issue, and the demands and capacities are not necessarily abnormal. Instead, it is the mismatch between the two that is the culprit. Treatment, then, is directed at increasing capacity in the face of an unchanged environment or decreasing environmental demands in the face of an unchanged capacity, or both—increasing capacity and decreasing demands. But such an explanation as that for stuttering is a tautology because it comes down to saying that a child stutters because he or she cannot be fluent within his or her communicative environment. Furthermore, the causative agent or agents cataloged by the model act linearly and unidirectionally: Increased capacity or decreased demand (or both) result in reduced stuttering. Neither the causative scenario explained by the model nor the treatment based on it reflects the notion that changes in capacity result from changes in environmental demand or that changes in environmental demand result from changes in capacity. As a model of etiology, the DCM suggests that stuttering results from a combination of constitutional factors categorized as capacity and environmental factors categorized as demands. Although the DCM implies that stuttering does not result from a single cause—children stutter not only because of constitutional factors but also because of the nature of the environment in which they communicate—the causative factors are static. That is, a given level of capacity and a given level of demand for a particular child will result in stuttering. Similarly, the DCM does not suggest that the demand and capacity factors actually interact with one another either to cause stuttering or to eliminate it. The reciprocal interaction of factors is the *sine qua non* of a transactional model and is inherent in the Lidcombe Program.

Principles of Effective Treatment

It is always exciting for me to discover connections and similarities between what appear to be different ideas or conceptualizations when they are viewed only superficially and separately. To discover those connections requires stepping out of one's specialty from time to time. So it is with the principles of effective treatment. I continue here with Hubbell's (1981) writing on the treatment of language disorders of children to show that the principles of effective treatment transcend disorder type. Hubbell (1981) posited six guiding principles for language intervention, five of which can be said to guide the intervention processes of the Lidcombe Program.

The first principle is that intervention must be ecologically valid. To be ecologically valid, treatment should be immediately functional for children in their daily lives. For language, this requires a focus on meaning and communication. For stuttering, this requires assistance to children for changing stuttered speech to stutter-free speech in the immediate context of structured and unstructured conversations.

The second principle is that intervention ought to take place through transactions. The point here is the same as that described previously in the section on the transactional model. Change occurs in the children and in their environments in reciprocal ways.

Hubbell (1981) takes the third principle from Moore and Anderson's work (as cited in Hubbell, 1981). Intervention should be autotelic in nature. Autotelic activities are those in which goals and rewards are intrinsic to the activities. These activities are engaged in for their own sake, and are enjoyable and appealing. The activities of verbal-contingent stimulation during structured and unstructured conversations have autotelic features. Recall the repeated statements of the contributors to this text that, by definition, the Lidcombe Program contingencies of praise, requests for correction of stuttering, and general verbal support are experienced by children as helpful and enjoyable.

The principle of autotelic activities is closely linked to the fourth principle of responsive environments, a concept also from the work of Moore and Anderson (as cited in Hubbell, 1981). A responsive environment provides learners with immediate feedback so that they know the consequences of their performance and can determine the rate at which events occur. Again, the Lidcombe Program's activities of contingent verbal stimulation during structured and unstructured conversations may be described as autotelic, responsive environments.

Exploratory teaching is the fifth principle that may be applied to the Lidcombe Program. The focus here is on the clinician and the parent who, through problem-solving strategies, change their behaviors to assist change in the children. The idea is to be responsive to children's individual needs and differences and to modify intervention accordingly.

Advice to Clinicians Who Might Worry: Don't

It has been my experience that clinicians unfamiliar with the Lidcombe Program, upon hearing that children are to be praised for nonstuttered speech and asked to correct stuttered speech, worry that things will be made worse by such procedures or, at the very least, that children will respond negatively. I suspect that these clinicians are still haunted by the ghost of the diagnosogenic theory. Any reluctance to treat early stuttering directly, however, will be erased once the information and procedures contained in this text are understood and once the data-based research on the program's efficacy, efficiency, and effectiveness is examined. Furthermore, it is important to note that response-contingent stimulation in the Lidcombe Program is not constant, intensive, or invasive, as stated explicitly in Chapters 6 and 8, and that children experience the program in positive and enjoyable ways. As explanations of the program's administration throughout the text make clear, treatment is planned and structured for each child individually. Because treatment is tailored to the individual child and because the program has the built-in safeguards described in the text (see Chapters 5 and 17), children are protected from the application or continuation of inappropriate or ineffective procedures.

What We Have Needed

I believe that the effective treatment of stuttering, in adults as well as in children, has been hampered by the paucity of structured, organized intervention programs that are both clinically useful and based on scientific evidence. By structured and organized, I do not mean programmed. I am not suggesting that the missing element has been programmed instruction. What I am suggesting is that treatment has all too often been based on amorphous assumptions and procedures that have been justified by wrapping them in the mantle of eclecticism. Eclecticism may have merit, but not when it results in scores of clinicians being presented with ill-defined or ambiguous treatment regimens during their academic and clinical training. That, unfortunately, has been the situation in stuttering treatment for many years. What have been needed are intervention programs that are based on organizing principles, that represent clearly articulated points of view, that are conceptually sound and evidence based, and that provide clinicians with direct guidance in the implementation of clinically useful methods and procedures. The Lidcombe Program and this Clinician's Guide meet those needs.

Simple or Complex?

It would be a disastrous mistake, however, to view either the Lidcombe Program or this guide as a cookbook or recipe book approach to the treatment of stuttering. The program and the guide are first and foremost conceptually based. This is not a one-size-fits-all treatment. Clinicians must decide what the appropriate treatment methods are for given clients. As Harrison, Trofari, Rousseau, and Andrews point out in Chapter 8, each application of the program is different because each child and family is different. Techniques and procedures are given meaning only when they are fitted to the individual and specific needs of the children who are to be treated.

One would be equally mistaken to come away from reading the text with the notion that the Lidcombe Program is simple in its conceptualization and administration. When I introduce the program to my graduate students, I warn them not to engage in that kind of self-deception. The program requires the intelligent application of its procedures to each child who is seen for evaluation or treatment. The unfolding of treatment for each child with whom the program is to be used will be different. The case studies presented in the text and the information on problem solving and troubleshooting are indications of the complexity of the program.

Indeed, the text makes it abundantly clear that the Lidcombe Program is not about the administration of response-contingent stimulation as the treatment agent (see Chapter 1) divorced from the context in which the children and their families live. The principles of sound clinical management familiar to and embraced by speech–language pathologists as best practice are found in the program. It would, therefore, be incorrect to characterize the program as strictly a behaviorist approach to the treatment of early stuttering. What the program and the concepts that drive it have done, however, is to rescue the management of stuttering from the pseudo-psychotherapeutic trap in which it has been held for so long and to acknowledge that the treatment of stuttering is not mysterious.

An example to illuminate this last point: When I was in Australia to observe the

Lidcombe Program firsthand, I had the opportunity to observe a clinician meeting with a child and his parents concerning the return of stuttering frequency to a formerly higher level. The child was in Stage 2 of the treatment. I can remember smiling to myself when I realized the direction in which the discussion was headed. Clinician and parents reviewed the program's purpose, components, strategies, and structure. The clinician assisted the parents in analyzing and then reemploying aspects of the program that would be expected to bring the frequency of stuttering down to the desired level. There were no discussions of family problems, school problems, or other sources of environmental stress as possible causative factors in the return of the child's stuttering. The focus was on how the parents might solve the problem within the context of the program. By the way, the child was in the room with the parents and clinician throughout the exchange. Later, when the clinician and I reviewed what took place during the session, I remarked on the absence of a discussion of possible environmental stress. The clinician simply reminded me of the nature of intervention for early stuttering on which the Lidcombe Program is based. This really is, I thought, an approach quite different from what we are accustomed to in the United States.

Is There a Theory Behind the Treatment?

If theory implies an explanation of cause and of treatment based on that cause, then theory will not be found in this text. The Lidcombe Program uses behavioral approaches that are based on operant methodology. The argument may be made that behaviorism and operant methodology are part of a theory of learning, but I suggest nevertheless that the program and the text are better viewed as being atheoretical. That suggestion is not meant to be a criticism. As Perkins (1986) has stated, theory may not be necessary for treatment to be effective. Furthermore, a scientific approach to stuttering intervention does not require that theory come first. The program is surely scientifically based and the text makes use of scientific principles throughout. The program's foundation is in the research that has investigated the operant properties of stuttering and in the work of those who have applied behavioral principles to the treatment of stuttering (Lincoln & Harrison, 1999).

Measurement Is the Rule

Yogi Berra, the great American baseball legend who has become equally famous for his quirky and funny one-liners known as Yogi-isms once said, "You've got to be careful if you don't know where you're going because you might not get there!" (Berra, 1998, p. 102). Yogi, of course, wasn't referring to measurement in stuttering intervention, but we can apply his unique logic to that issue nevertheless.

If we are to assess the progress children make in treatment and if we are to know whether they have reached the point where we can say that treatment has been successful and desired outcomes have been reached, then we had better establish the appropriate criteria. The Lidcombe Program, among other intervention programs, uses reductions in the severity and rate of stuttering as the metric for decision making throughout the course of treatment—measuring the initial severity of the stuttering, establishing goals, estimating progress, and moving from structured to unstructured treatment to maintenance. The within- and beyond-clinic measures described in the text are what enable clinicians to know where they and their clients are going and to know if they have gotten there. (Thanks Yogi.)

The use of quantitative and verifiable data in measuring treatment effects and in clinical reasoning is not merely desirable, it is mandatory. In the not too distant past, clinicians used vague and poorly defined criteria to make clinical judgments about stuttering and its management (Attanasio, 1999), and perhaps some clinicians continue to do so. The Lidcombe Program cannot be used without data-based measures; those measures are fundamental.

Timing of Intervention

I end this chapter by commenting on the questions of whether and when intervention for early stuttering should begin. Perhaps I have saved the thorniest issue for last. It is not my intention, however, to attempt a discussion of the many facets of timing intervention. The topic is amply discussed in Chapter 4. A few comments will do.

Although intervention for early stuttering is appropriate for many children (Attanasio, 1999) and although it is now clear that for great numbers of children—perhaps most—early stuttering is perceptually recognizable and distinguishable from nonstuttered disfluencies (Onslow, 1996), it is not axiomatic that all children who stutter should begin treatment as soon as they start to stutter. Nor is it axiomatic that no child should begin treatment as soon as the stuttering begins. It is important here to separate this issue of the timing of intervention from the issue of the identification of stuttering. Wrestling with the difficulties of deciding if and when to treat is not the same thing as deciding if a child is stuttering. The distinction is not a trivial one. It has been my experience that many clinicians make the decision not to treat because they are reluctant to or believe that they are unable to make a diagnosis of early stuttering. The decision not to treat is thereby made by default. This comes, I believe, from clinicians having been taught, mistakenly, that the diagnosis of early stuttering is difficult because it is not easy to distinguish early stuttering from the nonstuttered disfluency observed in the speech of many young children. The ghost of the diagnosogenic theory may also have had a role to play.

The concern with the timing of intervention has legitimately more to do with the real issue of natural recovery from stuttering (also described as spontaneous recovery or unaided recovery) than with anything else. That is the point of Chapter 4. It is readily seen in that chapter and in other commentary on the Lidcombe Program (Onslow & Packman, 1999) that the assessment of natural recovery in early stuttering is incorporated into the management strategies of the program. Rather than being made by default, the decision not to treat, if that is the decision reached, is an active one based on management strategy (Onslow & Packman, 1999).

I conclude this section and this chapter by making an admission that, if I were more prudent, I would not make. It is this: I wonder if we make more of the problem of natural recovery versus professional intervention than we should. After all, what would the real harm be if we took children who would have recovered from stuttering naturally into treatment? I recognize that professional ethics require that we not treat when treatment is unnecessary and that resources used to treat children who do not require our services are better allocated to children who do. As far as professional ethics are concerned, I argue that it is better to treat unnecessarily than to mistakenly withhold treatment from someone who needs it and that the only way to conclude that treatment was unnecessary for a particular child is to withhold treatment (at least for awhile) to see what happens. (I wonder what Yogi would say.) The resource problem, on the other hand, is a matter of economy, not a clinical management issue.

References

Attanasio, J. S. (1999). Treatment of early stuttering: Some reflections. In M. Onslow & A. Packman (Eds.), *The handbook of early stuttering intervention* (pp. 189–203). San Diego: Singular Publishing Group.

Attanasio, J. S. (2000). Where is the gap? A diverse view of stuttering and stuttering research [Review of the book *Stuttering research and practice: Bridging the gap*]. *Contemporary Psychology APA Review of Books*, *45*(1), 53–55.

Attanasio, J. S., Onslow, M., & Menzies, R. (1996). Australian and United States perspectives on stuttering in preschool children. *Australian Journal of Human Communication Disorders*, *24*, 55–61.

Berra, Y. (1998). *The Yogi book*. New York: Workman Publishing.

Culatta, R. (1976). Fluency: The other side of the coin. *Asha*, *18*, 795–799.

Hubbell, R. D. (1981). *Children's language disorders: An integrated approach*. Englewood Cliffs, NJ: Prentice Hall.

Lincoln, M., & Harrison, E. (1999). The Lidcombe Program. In M. Onslow & A. Packman (Eds.), *The handbook of early stuttering intervention* (pp. 103–117). San Diego: Singular Publishing Group.

Martin, R. R., Kuhl, P., & Haroldson, S. (1972). An experimental treatment with two preschool stuttering children. *Journal of Speech and Hearing Research*, *15*, 743–752.

Onslow, M. (1996). *Behavioral management of stuttering*. San Diego: Singular Publishing Group.

Onslow, M., Costa, L., & Rue, S. (1990). Direct early intervention with stuttering: Some preliminary data. *Journal of Speech and Hearing Disorders*, *55*, 405–416.

Onslow, M., & Packman, A. (1999). The Lidcombe Program and natural recovery: Potential choices of initial management strategies for early stuttering. *Advances in Speech–Language Pathology*, *1*, 113–121.

Perkins, W. H. (1986). Functions and malfunctions of theories in therapies. *Asha*, *28*, 31–33.

Prins, D., & Ingham, R. J. (Eds.). (1983). *Treatment of stuttering in early childhood: Methods and issues*. San Diego: College-Hill Press.

Index

About the Authors

Mark Onslow is director of the Australian Stuttering Research Centre at The University of Sydney. In addition to his academic appointment at The University of Sydney, he is an adjunct professor at the University of Canterbury, New Zealand. Mark's research interests are the nature and treatment of stuttering. He has taught university courses in stuttering management in three countries and currently teaches research methods to doctoral students at the Australian Stuttering Research Centre. Mark has published more than 100 articles in journals and conference proceedings. He has written a textbook on management of stuttering and with his colleague, Ann Packman, has edited a handbook on early stuttering intervention. He is in constant demand internationally as a speaker on the clinical management of stuttering.

Ann Packman is a researcher at the Australian Stuttering Research Centre, The University of Sydney. She has many years of experience in treatment and research with people who stutter. Ann has published many articles on stuttering in peer-reviewed journals and has presented widely at national and international conferences. In her current position, she is involved in a range of research projects on the nature and treatment of stuttering, and she supervises postgraduate research students. Ann is interested in theoretical issues in stuttering and is currently cowriting a text on this topic. Ann has been successful, with colleague Mark Onslow, in attracting funding for stuttering research from the Australian government.

Elisabeth Harrison has been the senior speech pathologist at the Stuttering Unit, Bankstown Health Service, Sydney, since 1990. The Stuttering Unit provides stuttering treatment for children and adults, as well as specialist consultation services for speech pathologists. The Stuttering Unit and the Australian Stuttering Research Centre, at The University of Sydney, collaborate in the conduct of clinical research about stuttering treatment. Together, staff from both organizations present professional development courses in stuttering treatment for clinicians. Elisabeth has conducted many workshops on stuttering treatment for speech pathologists in Australia, Canada, and the Netherlands. She has published many articles on stuttering in peer-reviewed journals. Elisabeth teaches a course in stuttering treatment in the speech pathology program at Macquarie University, Sydney.